Stay Young with Yoga

Discover How Practicing Yoga Can Help You Maintain Youthful Vitality and Flexibility throughout Your Lifetime

Lewis Finan

Table of Contents

Introduction:

In the quest for eternal youth, humans have traversed countless paths, from elixirs of legend to the latest advancements in skincare. Yet, amidst this cacophony of remedies, one ancient practice stands timeless and unwavering: yoga.

"Stay Young with Yoga: Discover How Practicing Yoga Can Help You Maintain Youthful Vitality and Flexibility throughout Your Lifetime" is an exploration of the profound connection between yoga and the fountain of youth. Within the serene confines of a yoga studio or the tranquil expanse of nature, individuals of all ages find solace, strength, and rejuvenation through the practice of yoga.

In a world perpetually in motion, where the demands of daily life often lead to physical and mental fatigue, yoga offers a sanctuary—a place where one can reconnect with the essence of youth, both in body and spirit. It is not merely a series of postures or breathwork; rather, yoga is a holistic journey towards holistic well-being, where each movement and each moment is an opportunity to cultivate vitality and flexibility.

Throughout the pages of this book, we will embark on a voyage through the rich tapestry of yoga, exploring its ancient roots, its modern manifestations, and its profound impact on the human body and mind. Drawing upon the wisdom of yogic philosophy and the latest scientific research, we will uncover the myriad ways in which yoga bestows its practitioners with the gifts of youthfulness: improved flexibility, enhanced vitality, heightened mental clarity, and a deep sense of inner peace.

Whether you are a seasoned yogi or a curious beginner, "Stay Young with Yoga" invites you to embark on a transformative journey—one that transcends the confines of age and time. Together, let us delve into the timeless teachings of yoga and discover how this ancient practice can empower you to embrace the fullness of life with grace, strength, and youthful vigor.

Chapter 1: The Fountain of Youth: Understanding the Benefits of Yoga

In the quest for eternal youth and vitality, humanity has traversed lands, sought elixirs, and delved into the depths of science. Yet, amidst this grand pursuit, one ancient practice stands timeless, offering profound rejuvenation not just for the body, but for the mind and spirit as well. Welcome to the wondrous world of yoga, where the fountain of youth flows ceaselessly, nourishing every facet of our being.

Origins of Yoga: A Tapestry of Tradition and Wisdom

To truly understand the essence of yoga, we must journey back through the annals of time to the ancient Indus Valley civilization, where the earliest traces of this transformative practice emerged. Rooted in the sacred texts of India, such as the Vedas and the Upanishads, yoga evolved as a holistic system for harmonizing the body, mind, and soul.

The word "yoga" itself stems from the Sanskrit term "yuj," meaning to yoke or unite, signifying the union of individual consciousness with the universal consciousness. Over millennia, yoga blossomed into a multifaceted discipline, encompassing various paths and practices, each designed to lead the seeker toward self-realization and inner peace.

The Yoga Renaissance: Embracing Ancient Wisdom in the Modern Age

In recent decades, there has been a remarkable resurgence of interest in yoga, fueled by a growing recognition of its profound benefits and supported by a burgeoning body of scientific research. From bustling metropolises to serene retreat centers, millions around the globe are embracing yoga as a means to enhance their physical health, mental well-being, and spiritual growth.

Physical Vitality: Strengthening the Temple of the Soul

At its core, yoga offers a holistic approach to physical fitness, cultivating strength, flexibility, and balance in the body. Through a dynamic interplay of asanas (physical postures), pranayama (breath control), and mindful movement, practitioners unlock the innate potential of their bodies, revitalizing muscles, joints, and organs.

Studies have shown that regular yoga practice can lead to numerous physiological benefits, including improved cardiovascular health, enhanced immune function, and reduced inflammation. Moreover, by fostering awareness of the body and its sensations, yoga empowers individuals to cultivate a deeper connection with their physical selves, fostering a sense of reverence and gratitude for the miraculous vessel that carries them through life.

Mental Clarity: Quieting the Turbulent Waters of the Mind

In today's fast-paced world, the mind often becomes a battleground of competing thoughts, emotions, and distractions, leading to stress, anxiety, and exhaustion. Yet, within the tranquil sanctuary of yoga, one discovers a refuge from the ceaseless chatter of the mind, a sacred space where stillness reigns supreme.

Through the practice of dhyana (meditation), mantra chanting, and mindfulness techniques, yoga cultivates mental clarity, emotional resilience, and inner peace. Scientific studies have elucidated the neurobiological mechanisms underlying these transformative effects, revealing how yoga modulates brain activity, promotes neuroplasticity, and enhances cognitive function.

Spiritual Awakening: Nurturing the Seed of Divinity Within

Beyond the realm of the physical and mental, yoga beckons us to embark on a profound journey of self-discovery and spiritual awakening. Rooted in the timeless wisdom of the sages, yoga invites us to transcend the limitations of ego and identity, awakening to the boundless expanses of our true nature.

Through practices such as self-inquiry, devotion (bhakti), and the cultivation of virtues such as compassion and equanimity, yoga guides us toward the realization of our inherent divinity, unveiling the eternal essence that animates all of creation. In this sacred union of the individual self with the universal Self, we discover the ultimate elixir of youth—the eternal spring of joy, love, and wisdom that flows ceaselessly within our hearts.

Embarking on the Journey: Embracing the Path of Yoga

As we stand on the threshold of this grand adventure, the path of yoga unfolds before us like a vast and wondrous tapestry, woven with threads of ancient wisdom and modern insight. Whether we are seasoned practitioners or curious novices, the journey of yoga invites us to embark with an open heart and a receptive mind, ready to embrace the transformative power of this timeless practice.

In the chapters that follow, we shall delve deeper into the rich tapestry of yoga, exploring its myriad paths, principles, and practices. From the gentle embrace of hatha yoga to the dynamic flow of vinyasa, from the devotional fervor of bhakti yoga to the introspective inquiry of jnana yoga, each facet of this multifaceted jewel offers its unique treasures, guiding us towards the realization of our highest potential.

So let us take the first step on this sacred journey, dear reader, as we embark together on the quest for the fountain of youth—the timeless essence of vitality, joy, and liberation that awaits us in the boundless depths of yoga's embrace.

1.1 Exploring the Origins of Yoga

To truly grasp the essence of yoga, we must embark on a journey through time to explore its origins deeply rooted in ancient civilizations. The history of yoga stretches back thousands of years, tracing its roots to the mystical lands of the Indus Valley, where the earliest evidence of yogic practices can be found.

Ancient Wisdom of the Indus Valley Civilization

The cradle of yoga lies nestled within the fertile plains of the ancient Indus Valley, a thriving civilization that flourished over 5,000 years ago in what is now present-day India and Pakistan. Among the ruins of Mohenjo-Daro and Harappa, archaeologist's unearthed seals depicting figures in yogic postures, offering tantalizing glimpses into the spiritual practices of this ancient culture.

The Vedas: Seeds of Yogic Wisdom

The sacred scriptures known as the Vedas, composed over 3,000 years ago, serve as the foundation upon which the edifice of yoga was erected. Within these revered texts, hymns and verses extol the virtues of meditation, self-discipline, and inner harmony, laying the groundwork for the yogic philosophy that would later blossom into a profound spiritual tradition.

The Upanishads: Illuminating the Path of Yoga

As the centuries unfolded, the wisdom of the Vedas found expression in the mystical teachings of the Upanishads, a collection of philosophical texts that delve into the nature of reality, the self, and the ultimate truths of existence. It is within the Upanishads that we encounter the concept of yoga as a means of realizing the union between individual consciousness (atman) and the universal consciousness (Brahman).

Sage Patanjali: Codifying the Yoga Sutras

In the second century BCE, the sage Patanjali distilled the essence of yogic wisdom into a systematic framework known as the Yoga Sutras. Comprising 196 aphorisms divided into four chapters, the Yoga Sutras delineate the path of Raja Yoga, or the royal path, which encompasses ethical precepts (yamas and niyamas), physical postures (asanas), breath control (pranayama), withdrawal of the senses (pratyahara), concentration (dharana), meditation (dhyana), and samadhi (union with the divine).

The Evolution of Yoga: Paths and Practices

Over the millennia, yoga underwent a process of evolution and diversification, giving rise to a multitude of paths and practices suited to the varied temperaments and aspirations of seekers. From the dynamic movements of hatha yoga to the devotional practices of bhakti yoga, from the intellectual inquiry of jnana yoga to the selfless service of karma yoga, each path offers its unique approach to realizing the timeless truths of yoga.

In tracing the origins of yoga, we unravel a rich tapestry woven from the threads of ancient wisdom and spiritual insight. From the sacred scriptures of the Vedas and Upanishads to the practical teachings of sage Patanjali, the journey of yoga spans the vast expanse of human history, offering a timeless path to self-discovery, inner peace, and spiritual liberation. As we delve deeper into the heart of yoga, let us honor the legacy of the sages and seekers who have illuminated this path before us, guiding us toward the eternal truths that lie at the core of our being.

1.2 Yoga Philosophy: Harmony of Body, Mind, and Spirit

At the heart of yoga lies a profound philosophy that embraces the unity of the body, mind, and spirit. Rooted in ancient wisdom and guided by timeless principles, yoga philosophy offers a holistic framework for understanding the nature of existence and the path to liberation.

The Five Koshas: Layers of Being

Central to yoga philosophy is the concept of the five koshas, or sheaths, which encapsulate the various dimensions of human existence:

- **Annamaya Kosha (Physical Sheath)**: The outermost layer comprises the physical body, including muscles, bones, and organs. Through the practice of asanas (physical postures) and pranayama (breath control), we cultivate strength, flexibility, and vitality in the physical sheath.
- **Pranamaya Kosha (Vital Sheath)**: Moving inward, we encounter the vital sheath, which encompasses the subtle energy that animates the physical body. Pranayama techniques harness the flow of prana, or life force energy, balancing and harmonizing the vital sheath.
- **Manomaya Kosha (Mental Sheath)**: Beyond the realm of the physical and energetic, we enter the domain of the mental sheath, which encompasses thoughts, emotions, and sensory perceptions. Through practices such as meditation and mindfulness, we cultivate awareness and clarity in the mental sheath.
- **Vijnanamaya Kosha (Wisdom Sheath)**: Deeper still lies the wisdom sheath, where intuitive knowledge and higher understanding reside. Through the cultivation of wisdom and

discernment, we gain insight into the true nature of reality and the self.

- **Anandamaya Kosha (Bliss Sheath)**: At the innermost core of our being lies the bliss sheath, which radiates with the divine joy and peace that transcends worldly concerns. Through the practice of self-realization and union with the divine, we awaken to the infinite bliss of our true nature.

The Eight Limbs of Yoga: Pathways to Liberation

In addition to the five koshas, yoga philosophy delineates the eight limbs of yoga, known as Ashtanga Yoga, as outlined by sage Patanjali in the Yoga Sutras. These limbs provide a comprehensive roadmap for spiritual growth and self-transformation:

- **Yamas (Ethical Restraints)**: Guidelines for ethical conduct towards oneself and others, including non-violence, truthfulness, non-stealing, moderation, and non-possessiveness.
- **Niyamas (Observances)**: Practices for self-discipline and inner purification, including cleanliness, contentment, self-discipline, self-study, and surrender to the divine.
- **Asanas (Physical Postures)**: Practices to cultivate strength, flexibility, and balance in the physical body, preparing the practitioner for deeper stages of meditation and self-realization.
- **Pranayama (Breath Control)**: Techniques to regulate the breath and vital energy, balancing the flow of prana and calming the fluctuations of the mind.

- **Pratyahara (Withdrawal of the Senses)**: Practices to turn inward and disengage from external distractions, fostering inner awareness and concentration.
- **Dharana (Concentration)**: The cultivation of focused attention on a single object or point, leading to deep states of absorption and meditation.
- **Dhyana (Meditation)**: The uninterrupted flow of awareness towards the chosen object of meditation, leading to profound states of inner stillness and self-realization.
- **Samadhi (Union with the Divine)**: The culmination of the yogic path, where the individual self merges with the universal consciousness, leading to the experience of pure bliss and liberation.

In essence, yoga philosophy serves as a guiding light on the journey of self-discovery and spiritual awakening. Through the integration of the five koshas and the eight limbs of yoga, we embark on a transformative quest to harmonize body, mind, and spirit, realizing the timeless truths of unity, peace, and liberation that lie at the core of our being. As we delve deeper into the teachings of yoga philosophy, may we find inspiration, guidance, and illumination on the path to wholeness and enlightenment.

1.3 Scientific Evidence: How Yoga Impacts Aging

In recent years, scientific research has increasingly recognized the profound impact of yoga on the aging process, shedding light on the mechanisms through which this ancient practice promotes physical health, mental well-being, and overall longevity. From enhancing flexibility and strength to reducing stress and inflammation, the benefits of yoga extend far beyond the confines of the yoga mat, offering a holistic approach to aging gracefully and vibrantly.

Physical Resilience: Strengthening the Body from Within

One of the most striking effects of yoga on aging is its ability to enhance physical resilience and vitality. Through a combination of asanas (physical postures), pranayama (breath control), and mindful movement, yoga improves flexibility, strength, and balance, thereby reducing the risk of falls, fractures, and age-related mobility issues.

Numerous studies have demonstrated the efficacy of yoga in improving functional fitness parameters such as muscle strength, joint flexibility, and aerobic capacity in older adults. By engaging in regular yoga practice, individuals can maintain and even enhance their physical capabilities, enabling them to lead active and independent lives well into their golden years.

Cognitive Function: Nurturing the Mind-Body Connection

In addition to its physical benefits, yoga exerts a profound influence on cognitive function and mental well-being. Through practices such as meditation, mindfulness, and breath awareness, yoga cultivates mental clarity, emotional resilience, and stress resilience, thereby mitigating the cognitive decline associated with aging.

Research has shown that yoga can enhance cognitive function in older adults, improving memory, attention, and executive function. Moreover, yoga has been found to modulate brain activity, promote neuroplasticity, and enhance connectivity within neural networks associated with memory, learning, and emotional regulation.

Stress Reduction: Balancing the Body's Stress Response

Chronic stress is a pervasive risk factor for accelerated aging and age-related diseases, contributing to inflammation, oxidative stress, and cellular damage. Yoga offers a potent antidote to stress, activating the body's relaxation response and promoting a state of calm and equanimity.

Studies have consistently demonstrated the efficacy of yoga in reducing stress levels and improving stress resilience in older adults. By practicing yoga regularly, individuals can lower levels of stress hormones such as cortisol, enhance heart rate variability, and cultivate a greater sense of well-being and emotional balance.

Inflammation: Alleviating Chronic Inflammatory Processes

Inflammation plays a central role in the aging process, contributing to the development of chronic diseases such as cardiovascular disease, diabetes, and neurodegenerative disorders. Yoga has emerged as a powerful tool for modulating inflammation, exerting anti-inflammatory effects at the cellular and molecular levels.

Research has shown that yoga can reduce markers of inflammation such as C-reactive protein (CRP), interleukin-6 (IL-6), and tumor necrosis factor-alpha (TNF-alpha) in older adults. By mitigating chronic low-grade inflammation, yoga helps to preserve tissue integrity, immune function, and overall healthspan, thereby promoting healthy aging from within.

In conclusion, the scientific evidence unequivocally supports the transformative potential of yoga in promoting healthy aging and enhancing the quality of life in older adults. From bolstering physical resilience and cognitive function to reducing stress and inflammation, yoga offers a multifaceted approach to aging gracefully and vibrantly.

As we continue to unravel the mysteries of yoga's impact on aging, may we embrace this ancient practice as a pathway to holistic well-being and longevity. By integrating yoga into our daily lives, we can cultivate vitality, resilience, and joy, empowering ourselves to age with grace, wisdom, and vitality.

Chapter 2: Embracing the Physical: Yoga Asanas for Strength and Flexibility

In the vibrant tapestry of yoga, the practice of asanas, or physical postures, serves as a cornerstone for cultivating strength, flexibility, and vitality in the body. From dynamic sequences that build heat and energy to gentle stretches that soothe and rejuvenate, yoga asanas offer a holistic approach to physical fitness that nourishes the body, mind, and spirit. In this chapter, we shall embark on a journey through the vast landscape of yoga asanas, exploring their myriad benefits and discovering how they can empower us to embrace the fullness of our physical potential.

The Power of Asanas: Harnessing the Body's Wisdom

At its essence, the practice of asanas is a celebration of the body's innate wisdom and intelligence. Through mindful movement and breath awareness, we awaken dormant energies, release tension, and unlock the boundless potential that resides within. Whether we are standing tall in Mountain Pose (Tadasana), flowing gracefully in Sun Salutations (Surya Namaskar), or surrendering into the restorative embrace of Child's Pose (Balasana), each asana invites us to explore the intricate interplay of strength and flexibility, stability and surrender, effort and ease.

Building Strength: Foundations for Stability and Resilience

Strength forms the bedrock of physical well-being, providing stability, support, and resilience in the face of life's challenges. In yoga, we cultivate strength not through brute force or aggression, but through mindful engagement, alignment, and breathe awareness. By integrating principles of alignment and muscle engagement, we build functional strength that extends beyond the confines of the yoga mat, empowering us to move with grace and confidence in our daily lives.

Warrior Poses: Embodying Courage and Determination

The Warrior poses—Warrior I (Virabhadrasana I), Warrior II (Virabhadrasana II), and Warrior III (Virabhadrasana III)—invite us to embody the qualities of courage, determination, and resilience. Rooted firmly into the earth, we stretch our arms wide, gaze steadfastly ahead, and sink deep into the lunge, cultivating strength in the legs, stability in the core, and openness in the heart. With each breath, we tap into the warrior spirit that resides within, empowering us to face life's challenges with grace and fortitude.

Plank Pose: Cultivating Core Stability and Inner Strength

In Plank Pose (Phalakasana), we harness the power of the core muscles to create a stable and strong foundation. With hands firmly planted on the mat and toes tucked under, we engage the abdominal muscles, lift the hips, and extend the spine, creating a straight line from head to heels. As we hold this pose with steady breath and focused awareness, we cultivate core stability, upper body strength, and mental resilience, preparing us to navigate the ebb and flow of life with poise and strength.

Cultivating Flexibility: Embracing Fluidity and Adaptability

Flexibility is the hallmark of a healthy and vibrant body, allowing for freedom of movement, ease of function, and a sense of spaciousness within. In yoga, we cultivate flexibility not only in the muscles and joints but also in the mind and heart, fostering a sense of openness, receptivity, and adaptability to life's ever-changing rhythms. Through gentle stretches, deep breathing, and mindful awareness, we unravel the layers of tension that bind us, inviting us to expand into the fullness of our being.

Forward Folds: Surrendering and Letting Go

Forward folds such as Uttanasana (Standing Forward Bend) and Paschimottanasana (Seated Forward Bend) offer a profound opportunity to surrender, release, and let go. With each exhalation, we melt forward from the hips, lengthening the spine, and surrendering the weight of the head and torso towards the earth. As we soften into the pose, we release tension in the hamstrings, lower back, and shoulders, inviting a sense of deep relaxation and renewal. With each breath, we cultivate a spirit of surrender and acceptance, allowing ourselves to flow with the rhythm of life's unfolding.

Hip Openers: Embracing Vulnerability and Release

Hip-opening poses such as Pigeon Pose (Eka Pada Rajakapotasana) and Cow Face Pose (Gomukhasana) invite us to explore the intricate terrain of the hips, pelvis, and groin. As we sink into these deep stretches, we encounter not only physical resistance but also emotional and energetic blockages stored within the hip region. With each breath, we gently coax the hips open, releasing stagnant energy, and inviting a sense of freedom, fluidity, and emotional release. In the spaciousness of the hips, we find a gateway to deeper layers of self-awareness, healing, and transformation.

In the grand dance of life, strength and flexibility are not opposing forces but complementary aspects of our embodied existence. Through the practice of yoga asanas, we learn to harmonize these qualities within ourselves, cultivating a balanced and integrated approach to physical fitness and well-being. As we continue to explore the vast landscape of yoga asanas, may we embrace the fullness of our physical potential, embodying strength, flexibility, and grace in every aspect of our lives.

2.1 Gentle Yoga Poses for Beginners

Yoga is a journey of self-discovery and transformation, accessible to practitioners of all ages, backgrounds, and fitness levels. For beginners seeking to embark on this sacred journey, gentle yoga poses offer a nurturing and supportive introduction to the practice, allowing for exploration, relaxation, and inner peace. In this section, we shall explore a selection of gentle yoga poses that are ideal for beginners, fostering a sense of grounding, flexibility, and well-being in both body and mind.

1. Mountain Pose (Tadasana)

Benefits: Mountain Pose serves as a foundation for many standing poses, helping to improve posture, alignment, and balance. It also promotes a sense of grounding and stability.

How to Practice:

- Stand tall with your feet hip-width apart, toes pointing forward, and arms relaxed by your sides.
- Engage your thighs, lengthen your spine, and lift your chest.
- Press firmly into the ground through your feet, feeling rooted and grounded like a mountain.
- Gaze softly ahead and breathe deeply, allowing your body to relax and your mind to become calm and centered.

2. Cat-Cow Stretch (Marjaryasana-Bitilasana)

Benefits: Cat-Cow Stretch gently warms up the spine, improves spinal flexibility, and releases tension in the back, neck, and shoulders. It also promotes awareness of breath and movement.

How to Practice:

- Begin on your hands and knees in a tabletop position, with your wrists aligned under your shoulders and your knees under your hips.
- Inhale as you arch your back, lifting your chest and tailbone towards the ceiling (Cow Pose).
- Exhale as you round your back, tucking your chin to your chest and drawing your belly button towards your spine (Cat Pose).
- Continue flowing between Cow Pose and Cat Pose with each inhale and exhale, moving at your own pace and focusing on the rhythm of your breath.

3. Child's Pose (Balasana)

Benefits: Child's Pose gently stretches the spine, hips, and thighs, while also promoting relaxation and stress relief. It provides a soothing counterpose to more active yoga poses.

How to Practice:

- Kneel on the mat with your big toes touching and knees hip-width apart.
- Sit back on your heels and extend your arms forward, lowering your forehead to the mat.
- Rest your arms alongside your body or extend them forward, palms facing down.
- Breathe deeply into your back body, feeling a gentle stretch in your spine and hips.
- Stay in Child's Pose for several breaths, allowing yourself to surrender and release tension with each exhale.

4. Seated Forward Bend (Paschimottanasana)

Benefits: Seated Forward Bend stretches the entire back body, including the spine, hamstrings, and calves. It also calms the mind and promotes introspection and relaxation.

How to Practice:

- Sit on the mat with your legs extended in front of you, feet flexed and toes pointing towards the ceiling.
- Inhale as you lengthen your spine and lift your arms overhead.
- Exhale as you hinge forward from the hips, reaching towards your feet with your hands.
- Keep your spine long and your chest open, folding forward with each exhale.
- Hold the stretch for several breaths, relaxing into the pose and allowing your body to soften and release.

5. Supine Twist (Supta Matsyendrasana)

Benefits: Supine Twist gently stretches the spine, shoulders, and hips, while also massaging the abdominal organs and promoting detoxification. It helps to release tension and improve spinal mobility.

How to Practice:

- Lie on your back with your arms extended out to the sides, palms facing down.
- Bend your knees and bring them towards your chest.
- Exhale as you lower your knees to the right side of your body, keeping both shoulders grounded.
- Turn your head to the left and gaze towards your left hand.
- Breathe deeply into the twist, feeling a gentle stretch in your spine and hips.

- Repeat on the other side, lowering your knees to the left and turning your head to the right.

As beginners on the path of yoga, these gentle poses offer a welcoming invitation to explore the body, breath, and mind with curiosity and compassion. Whether practiced individually or woven together in a flowing sequence, these poses provide a safe and nurturing foundation for building strength, flexibility, and inner peace. As you journey deeper into the practice, may these gentle yoga poses serve as trusted companions, guiding you towards greater health, happiness, and self-discovery.

2.2 Intermediate Asanas to Build Strength

As your yoga practice evolves and your body grows stronger, intermediate asanas offer an opportunity to deepen your physical capabilities, challenge your limits, and cultivate a greater sense of power and resilience. In this section, we will explore a selection of intermediate yoga poses that focus on building strength in key areas of the body, including the core, arms, legs, and back. These poses will help you develop stability, balance, and muscular endurance, enabling you to progress confidently on your journey toward physical mastery and inner transformation.

1. Boat Pose (Navasana)

Benefits: Boat Pose strengthens the core muscles, including the abdominals, hip flexors, and lower back. It also improves balance, posture, and concentration.

How to Practice:

- Begin seated on the mat with your knees bent and feet flat on the floor, hands resting on the thighs.
- Lean back slightly and lift your feet off the floor, balancing on your sit bones.
- Extend your legs forward, keeping them together and parallel to the floor.
- Reach your arms forward alongside your legs, palms facing each other.
- Engage your core muscles and lift your chest, lengthening your spine.
- Hold the pose for several breaths, maintaining a strong and steady posture.

2. Side Plank Pose (Vasisthasana)

Benefits: Side Plank Pose strengthens the arms, wrists, core, and legs, while also improving balance and coordination. It targets the obliques and lateral muscles of the torso.

How to Practice:

- Begin in Plank Pose, with your wrists aligned under your shoulders and your body forming a straight line from head to heels.
- Shift your weight onto your right hand and the outer edge of your right foot, stacking your left foot on top of the right.

- Lift your left arm towards the ceiling, extending it straight overhead or placing it on your hip for support.
- Engage your core muscles and lift your hips, creating a straight line from head to heels.
- Hold the pose for several breaths, maintaining stability and alignment.
- Repeat on the other side, shifting your weight to your left hand and the outer edge of your left foot.

3. Warrior III Pose (Virabhadrasana III)

Benefits: Warrior III Pose strengthens the legs, core, and back muscles, while also improving balance, focus, and coordination. It cultivates a sense of groundedness and stability.

How to Practice:

- Begin in Mountain Pose (Tadasana), standing tall with your feet hip-width apart and arms by your sides.
- Shift your weight onto your right foot and hinge forward at the hips, extending your left leg straight back behind you.
- Keep your hips level and your torso parallel to the floor, reaching your arms forward alongside your ears or placing your hands on your hips for support.
- Engage your core muscles and press firmly through your standing foot, lifting your left leg higher and extending through the heel.
- Lengthen your spine and gaze forward, finding a focal point to help you maintain balance.

- Hold the pose for several breaths, then switch sides, balancing on your left foot and extending your right leg back.

4. Dolphin Pose (Ardha Pincha Mayurasana)

Benefits: Dolphin Pose strengthens the arms, shoulders, core, and legs, while also stretching the spine and hamstrings. It improves upper body strength and stability.

How to Practice:

- Begin on your hands and knees in Tabletop Pose, with your wrists aligned under your shoulders and your knees under your hips.
- Lower onto your forearms, placing your elbows directly under your shoulders and interlacing your fingers.
- Tuck your toes under and lift your hips towards the ceiling, straightening your legs and forming an inverted V shape with your body.
- Press firmly into your forearms and hands, engaging your core muscles and lifting your sit bones towards the ceiling.
- Keep your neck relaxed and gaze towards your feet, allowing your heels to sink towards the floor.
- Hold the pose for several breaths, feeling a deep stretch in the shoulders, hamstrings, and spine.

5. Crow Pose (Bakasana)

Benefits: Crow Pose strengthens the arms, wrists, core, and hip flexors, while also improving balance, focus, and coordination. It cultivates courage and confidence.

How to Practice:

- Begin in a squat position with your feet hip-width apart and your knees bent, placing your hands shoulder-width apart on the mat in front of you.
- Shift your weight onto your hands, bending your elbows slightly and leaning forward.
- Lift your hips high, bringing your knees towards your upper arms or armpits, and engaging your core muscles.
- Gaze forward and shift your weight onto your hands, lifting your feet off the floor one at a time.
- Balance on your hands, pressing firmly into the mat with your fingertips and engaging your abdominal muscles.
- Hold the pose for several breaths, focusing on stability and strength, then gently release back to the mat.

As you incorporate these intermediate yoga poses into your practice, remember to approach them with patience, mindfulness, and respect for your body's capabilities. With consistent practice and dedication, you will gradually build strength, flexibility, and resilience, both on and off the mat. As you deepen your physical practice, may you also cultivate a greater sense of inner strength, courage, and self-awareness, empowering you to navigate life's challenges with grace and confidence.

2.3 Advanced Yoga Postures to Enhance Flexibility

Advanced yoga postures offer an opportunity to explore the outer limits of your physical capabilities, challenging your flexibility, strength, and balance in profound ways. In this section, we will delve into a selection of advanced yoga poses that focus specifically on enhancing flexibility throughout the body. These poses require a high degree of strength, mobility, and body awareness, and should only be attempted by experienced practitioners who have developed a solid foundation in yoga practice. As you embark on this journey, approach these poses with patience, mindfulness, and respect for your body's limitations, honoring the wisdom of your unique practice.

1. King Pigeon Pose (Kapotasana)

Benefits: King Pigeon Pose deeply stretches the hip flexors, quadriceps, and chest, while also improving spinal mobility and shoulder flexibility. It opens the heart center and cultivates emotional release and surrender.

How to Practice:

- Begin in Downward Facing Dog Pose (Adho Mukha Svanasana), with your hands shoulder-width apart and your feet hip-width apart.
- Step your right foot forward between your hands and lower your left knee to the mat.
- Slide your right foot over towards your left hand, bringing your knee towards your right hand.

- Reach back with your left hand to grab your left foot or ankle, drawing it towards your body.
- Press into your right hand and lift your chest towards the sky, arching your back and opening your heart.
- Hold the pose for several breaths, then repeat on the other side.

2. Standing Split Pose (Urdhva Prasarita Eka Padasana)

Benefits: Standing Split Pose stretches the hamstrings, calves, and hip flexors, while also improving balance, coordination, and concentration. It strengthens the legs and core muscles.

How to Practice:

- Begin in Mountain Pose (Tadasana), standing tall with your feet together and arms by your sides.
- Shift your weight onto your left foot and lift your right leg straight up towards the ceiling, flexing the foot.
- Keep your hips squared towards the front of the mat and your torso parallel to the floor.
- Extend through the crown of your head and reach your fingertips towards the floor, framing your standing foot.
- Flex your left foot and engage your quadriceps to stabilize the standing leg.
- Hold the pose for several breaths, then gently release and repeat on the other side.

3. Compass Pose (Parivrtta Surya Yantrasana)

Benefits: Compass Pose deeply stretches the hamstrings, outer hips, and shoulders, while also improving spinal mobility and core strength. It challenges balance and coordination.

How to Practice:

- Begin seated on the mat with your legs extended in front of you.
- Bend your right knee and bring the sole of your right foot to the floor, close to your right sit bone.
- Reach your right arm behind your back and clasp your right big toe with your left hand.
- Extend your left arm forward and hook your left foot with your right hand.
- Flex both feet and engage your quadriceps to straighten both legs.
- Extend through the crown of your head and lift your chest towards the sky, twisting gently to the left.
- Hold the pose for several breaths, then gently release and repeat on the other side.

4. Monkey Pose (Hanumanasana)

Benefits: Monkey Pose deeply stretches the hamstrings, quadriceps, and hip flexors, while also improving hip mobility and flexibility. It cultivates patience, perseverance, and surrender.

How to Practice:

- Begin in a low lunge position with your right foot forward and your left knee on the mat.
- Walk your right foot forward and straighten your right leg, flexing the foot.
- Slide your left knee back and your right foot forward until your hips are square and your legs are straight.
- Place your hands on the floor or blocks for support, framing your right foot.
- Engage your quadriceps and press firmly through your right heel to activate the stretch.
- Lengthen through the spine and lift your chest towards the sky, finding a gentle backbend.
- Hold the pose for several breaths, then gently release and repeat on the other side.

5. Eight-Angle Pose (Astavakrasana)

Benefits: Eight-Angle Pose strengthens the arms, wrists, core, and legs, while also improving balance, concentration, and coordination. It challenges the practitioner to find stability and ease in a complex arm balance.

How to Practice:

- Begin seated on the mat with your legs extended in front of you.

- Bend your knees and place your hands on the mat behind your hips, fingers pointing towards your feet.
- Lean back slightly and lift your hips off the mat, engaging your core muscles.
- Bend your elbows and shift your weight onto your hands, lifting your feet off the floor.
- Cross your right ankle over your left thigh, hooking your right foot behind your left calf.
- Extend your left leg straight out to the side, parallel to the floor.
- Press firmly into your hands and engage your core to lift your hips higher.
- Hold the pose for several breaths, then gently release and repeat on the other side.

As you explore these advanced yoga postures, remember to approach them with humility, mindfulness, and respect for your body's limitations. Flexibility is not just about physical suppleness, but also about cultivating an open mind, a compassionate heart, and a resilient spirit. With consistent practice and dedication, you will gradually deepen your flexibility, strength, and self-awareness, both on and off the mat. As you journey deeper into the practice, may you continue to embrace the challenges and blessings of the path with grace, courage, and unwavering determination.

Chapter 3: Nurturing the Mind: Yoga for Mental Well-being

In the fast-paced and often chaotic world we live in, nurturing our mental well-being is essential for maintaining a sense of balance, resilience, and inner peace. Yoga offers a profound pathway to cultivate mental clarity, emotional resilience, and a deep sense of inner calm. In this chapter, we will explore the transformative power of yoga for nurturing the mind, offering practices and techniques that promote mental well-being, emotional balance, and spiritual growth.

The Mind-Body Connection: Uniting Body, Breath, and Mind

At the heart of yoga lies the recognition of the intimate connection between the body, breath, and mind. Through the practice of asanas (physical postures), pranayama (breath control), and meditation, we learn to synchronize our movements with our breath and cultivate a deep awareness of the present moment. This integration of body, breath, and mind forms the foundation for nurturing mental well-being and fostering a sense of inner harmony and balance.

Cultivating Mindfulness: The Art of Presence

Central to the practice of yoga for mental well-being is the cultivation of mindfulness—the art of being fully present in the moment, with an open heart and non-judgmental awareness. Mindfulness allows us to observe our thoughts, emotions, and sensations with curiosity and compassion, without getting entangled in their stories or judgments. Through mindfulness practices such as mindful breathing, body scans, and loving-kindness meditation, we develop greater self-awareness, emotional regulation, and resilience in the face of life's challenges.

Stress Reduction: Finding Stillness amid Chaos

Chronic stress is a pervasive threat to our mental and emotional well-being, contributing to anxiety, depression, and burnout. Yoga offers a sanctuary of stillness amidst the chaos of daily life, providing tools and techniques to soothe the nervous system, quiet the mind, and release accumulated tension and stress. Practices such as restorative yoga, yoga nidra, and guided relaxation promote deep relaxation and rejuvenation, allowing the body and mind to heal and restore balance.

Emotional Healing: Embracing the Full Spectrum of Feelings

Emotions are a natural and essential part of the human experience, yet many of us struggle to navigate the complexities of our inner world. Yoga offers a safe and supportive space to explore and embrace the full spectrum of emotions, from joy and gratitude to sadness and grief. Through practices such as heart-opening poses, journaling, and self-inquiry, we learn to cultivate greater emotional awareness, acceptance, and resilience, allowing us to move through life with greater grace and authenticity.

Cultivating Compassion: The Heart of Yoga

At the heart of yoga for mental well-being lies the practice of compassion—both towards ourselves and others. Compassion is the antidote to self-criticism, judgment, and isolation, offering a pathway to healing, connection, and inner peace. Through practices such as metta (loving-kindness) meditation, seva (selfless service), and acts of kindness towards ourselves and others, we cultivate a sense of interconnectedness and belonging, fostering a more compassionate and inclusive world for all beings.

As we journey deeper into the practice of yoga for mental well-being, may we remember that the true essence of yoga lies not in achieving perfection or attaining external goals, but in the journey of self-discovery and transformation. Through the integration of body, breath, and mind, may we cultivate greater self-awareness, emotional resilience, and inner peace, empowering ourselves to navigate life's challenges with grace, wisdom, and compassion. As we walk this path together, may we support and uplift one another, knowing that we are all interconnected and deserving of love, acceptance, and belonging.

3.1 Yoga Breathing Techniques for Stress Reduction

Yoga offers a treasure trove of breathing techniques, known as pranayama, that serve as powerful tools for reducing stress, calming the mind, and promoting overall well-being. By harnessing the breath, we can tap into the body's innate relaxation response, activating the parasympathetic nervous system and inducing a state of calm and tranquility. In this section, we will explore several yoga breathing techniques that are particularly effective for stress reduction, offering simple yet potent practices that can be incorporated into your daily routine.

1. Deep Belly Breathing (Diaphragmatic Breathing)

Benefits: Deep belly breathing activates the diaphragm, the primary muscle of respiration, and promotes relaxation by engaging the parasympathetic nervous system. It helps to reduce stress, anxiety, and tension in the body and mind.

How to Practice:

- Find a comfortable seated or lying position, with your spine tall and your shoulders relaxed.
- Place one hand on your chest and the other hand on your abdomen.
- Inhale deeply through your nose, allowing your abdomen to expand as you fill your lungs with air.
- Exhale slowly and completely through your nose or mouth, drawing your navel towards your spine.
- Continue to breathe deeply into your belly, feeling it rise and fall with each breath.
- Practice for several minutes, allowing yourself to relax and let go with each exhalation.

2. Equal Breathing (Sama Vritti Pranayama)

Benefits: Equal breathing balances the flow of prana (life force energy) in the body and calms the mind. It promotes focus, clarity, and emotional stability, making it an excellent practice for reducing stress and anxiety.

How to Practice:

- Find a comfortable seated position or lie down on your back with your spine straight.
- Inhale deeply through your nose for a count of four.
- Exhale slowly and evenly through your nose for a count of four.
- Continue to inhale and exhale for the same count, maintaining a smooth and steady rhythm.
- As you become more comfortable with the practice, you can gradually increase the count to six, eight, or even ten.
- Practice for several minutes, allowing your breath to anchor you in the present moment.

3. Alternate Nostril Breathing (Nadi Shodhana Pranayama)

Benefits: Alternate nostril breathing balances the flow of prana in the body, harmonizes the left and right hemispheres of the brain, and calms the nervous system. It reduces stress, anxiety, and mental agitation, promoting a sense of inner balance and peace.

How to Practice:

- Find a comfortable seated position with your spine tall and your shoulders relaxed.
- Use your right thumb to close your right nostril and inhale deeply through your left nostril for a count of four.
- Close your left nostril with your right ring finger, and hold your breath for a count of four.
- Release your right thumb and exhale slowly and evenly through your right nostril for a count of four.
- Inhale deeply through your right nostril for a count of four.
- Close your right nostril with your right thumb, and hold your breath for a count of four.
- Release your left ring finger and exhale slowly and evenly through your left nostril for a count of four.
- Continue to alternate nostrils with each breath, maintaining a smooth and steady rhythm.
- Practice for several minutes, allowing the breath to calm and center you.

4. Victorious Breath (Ujjayi Pranayama)

Benefits: Victorious breath creates a soothing sound by slightly constricting the back of the throat, which calms the mind and reduces stress. It promotes relaxation, concentration, and mental clarity, making it an excellent practice for stress reduction and meditation.

How to Practice:

- Find a comfortable seated position with your spine tall and your shoulders relaxed.
- Inhale deeply through your nose, drawing the breath in through the back of your throat to create a soft hissing sound.
- Exhale slowly and evenly through your nose, continuing to gently constrict the throat to create the same sound.
- Keep the breath smooth and steady, with each inhale and exhale of equal length.
- As you become more comfortable with the practice, you can gradually increase the length of your inhalations and exhalations.
- Practice for several minutes, allowing the sound of your breath to anchor you in the present moment.

As you incorporate these yoga breathing techniques into your daily routine, remember that the breath is a powerful ally on your journey towards stress reduction and inner peace. By cultivating awareness and mindfulness of the breath, you can tap into a deep reservoir of calm and resilience, even amid life's challenges. Whether you practice deep belly breathing, equal breathing, alternate nostril breathing, or victorious breath, may each breath serve as a reminder of your innate capacity for relaxation, clarity, and well-being.

3.2 Meditation Practices for Clarity and Focus

Meditation is a time-honored practice that offers a sanctuary of stillness amidst the chaos of daily life. By cultivating mindfulness and concentration, meditation promotes clarity, focus, and inner peace, empowering us to navigate life's challenges with grace and resilience. In this section, we will explore several meditation practices that are specifically designed to enhance clarity and focus, providing tools and techniques to quiet the mind, sharpen our awareness, and awaken to the present moment.

1. Mindfulness Meditation

Benefits: Mindfulness meditation cultivates present-moment awareness and non-judgmental observation of thoughts, emotions, and sensations. It promotes clarity, insight, and emotional balance, making it an effective practice for reducing stress, anxiety, and mental agitation.

How to Practice:

- Find a comfortable seated position with your spine tall and your shoulders relaxed.
- Close your eyes or soften your gaze, allowing your attention to turn inward.
- Bring your awareness to the sensations of your breath, noticing the rise and fall of your abdomen or the sensation of air passing through your nostrils.

- As thoughts, emotions, or sensations arise, simply observe them without judgment or attachment, allowing them to come and go like clouds passing through the sky.
- Whenever you notice your mind wandering, gently bring your attention back to the breath, anchoring yourself in the present moment.
- Practice for several minutes, gradually increasing the duration as you become more comfortable with the practice.

2. Focused Attention Meditation

Benefits: Focused attention meditation trains the mind to sustain attention on a single object or point of focus, such as the breath, a mantra, or a visual image. It enhances concentration, mental clarity, and cognitive function, making it an excellent practice for improving productivity and performance.

How to Practice:

- Choose a point of focus for your meditation, such as the sensation of your breath at the nostrils, the sound of a mantra, or a visual object placed in front of you.
- Settle into a comfortable seated position with your spine tall and your shoulders relaxed.
- Direct your attention to your chosen point of focus, allowing all other thoughts and distractions to fade into the background.
- If your mind wanders, gently and non-judgmentally bring your attention back to your chosen focal point, recommitting to the practice of sustained attention.

- Maintain your focus for the duration of the meditation, allowing yourself to sink deeper into a state of concentration and absorption.
- Practice for several minutes, gradually increasing the duration as you strengthen your ability to sustain attention.

3. Body Scan Meditation

Benefits: Body scan meditation involves systematically scanning through the body with mindful awareness, bringing attention to each area and noticing any sensations that arise. It promotes relaxation, body awareness, and emotional balance, making it an effective practice for reducing stress and tension.

How to Practice:

- Find a comfortable lying position on your back, with your arms by your sides and your legs extended.
- Close your eyes and take a few deep breaths, allowing your body to relax and settle into the mat.
- Begin at the top of your head and bring your awareness to the sensations in your scalp, forehead, and face. Notice any areas of tension or relaxation.
- Slowly move your awareness down through your body, scanning each area in turn, including the neck, shoulders, chest, arms, hands, abdomen, pelvis, legs, and feet.
- As you scan through each area, observe any sensations that arise, such as warmth, tingling, or pressure, without trying to change or manipulate them.

- If you encounter areas of tension or discomfort, bring your breath into that area and imagine it softening and releasing with each exhale.
- Continue scanning through your entire body, from head to toe, until you reach a state of deep relaxation and presence.
- Practice for several minutes, allowing yourself to rest in the spaciousness of your awareness.

4. Visualization Meditation

Benefits: Visualization meditation involves mentally imagining a peaceful, serene, or uplifting scene, such as a beach, forest, or mountaintop. It promotes relaxation, stress reduction, and positive mood, making it an effective practice for enhancing mental clarity and focus.

How to Practice:

- Find a comfortable seated or lying position with your eyes closed.
- Take a few deep breaths to relax your body and quiet your mind.
- Begin to visualize a scene that brings you a sense of peace, tranquility, or joy. This could be a place in nature, a favorite vacation spot, or a peaceful sanctuary within your imagination.
- Engage all of your senses in the visualization, imagining the sights, sounds, smells, textures, and sensations of your chosen scene.
- Allow yourself to fully immerse in the experience, feeling yourself becoming more relaxed, calm, and present with each breath.

- If your mind wanders, gently bring your attention back to the visualization, refocusing on the details and sensations of your imagined scene.
- Continue to visualize for several minutes, allowing yourself to rest in the beauty and tranquility of your inner landscape.

As you explore these meditation practices for clarity and focus, remember that the essence of meditation lies not in achieving a particular state of mind, but in the journey of self-discovery and self-awareness. Each moment of presence, each breath of awareness, is an opportunity to awaken to the fullness of life unfolding within and around you. Whether you choose to practice mindfulness meditation, focused attention meditation, body scan meditation, or visualization meditation, may each moment of meditation bring you closer to the clarity, focus, and inner peace that reside at the heart of your being.

3.3 Yoga Nidra: The Art of Deep Relaxation

Yoga Nidra, often referred to as "yogic sleep," is a powerful meditation technique that induces a state of deep relaxation and profound inner awareness. Rooted in ancient yogic wisdom, Yoga Nidra guides practitioners into a state of conscious relaxation, where the body and mind can rest deeply while remaining fully awake and aware. In this section, we will explore the practice of Yoga Nidra and its transformative benefits for physical, mental, and emotional well-being.

Understanding Yoga Nidra

Yoga Nidra is a systematic practice that guides practitioners through a series of stages, leading to a state of deep relaxation and inner stillness. The practice typically begins with a body scan, where attention is directed to different parts of the body, systematically releasing tension and promoting relaxation. This is followed by a rotation of awareness through various sensations, feelings, and emotions, allowing practitioners to observe and witness their inner experiences without judgment or attachment. Finally, the practice concludes with the setting of an intention, known as a Sankalpa, which is a positive affirmation or statement of purpose that aligns with the practitioner's deepest desires and aspirations.

Benefits of Yoga Nidra

Yoga Nidra offers a wide range of benefits for physical, mental, and emotional well-being, including:

- **Stress Reduction**: By inducing a state of deep relaxation, Yoga Nidra helps to reduce levels of stress hormones in the body, promoting a sense of calm and tranquility.
- **Improved Sleep**: Regular practice of Yoga Nidra can help to improve sleep quality and alleviate insomnia, allowing practitioners to experience more restful and rejuvenating sleep.
- **Enhanced Creativity and Focus**: By quieting the mind and promoting mental clarity, Yoga Nidra can enhance creativity, concentration, and focus, enabling practitioners to tap into their inner wisdom and insight.

- **Emotional Healing**: Through the practice of witnessing and observing inner experiences without judgment, Yoga Nidra can facilitate emotional healing and release, allowing practitioners to process and integrate challenging emotions with greater ease.
- **Self-Discovery and Self-Realization**: Yoga Nidra offers a pathway to self-discovery and self-realization, allowing practitioners to connect with their true essence and tap into the limitless potential within.

How to Practice Yoga Nidra

To practice Yoga Nidra, follow these simple steps:

- Find a Comfortable Position: Lie down on your back in Savasana (Corpse Pose), with your arms by your sides, palms facing up, and legs extended comfortably.
- Set an Intention: Take a moment to reflect on your intention or Sankalpa for the practice. This could be a positive affirmation or statement of purpose that aligns with your deepest desires and aspirations.
- Relax the Body: Close your eyes and take a few deep breaths to relax your body and mind. Begin to bring awareness to different parts of your body, starting with your toes and moving up through your legs, torso, arms, and head. Allow each part of your body to relax and release tension as you bring attention to it.
- Rotate Awareness: After relaxing the body, begin to rotate your awareness through different sensations, feelings, and emotions. Notice any sensations of warmth, heaviness, or tingling in different

parts of your body. Observe any thoughts, emotions, or memories that arise, allowing them to come and go without attachment.

- Repeat Your Intention: Towards the end of the practice, return to your intention or Sankalpa, repeating it silently to yourself three times with conviction and clarity.
- Transition Back to Waking Consciousness: Gradually bring your awareness back to your surroundings, gently wiggle your fingers and toes, and take a few deep breaths. When you feel ready, slowly open your eyes and sit up slowly.

As you explore the practice of Yoga Nidra, remember that the true essence of the practice lies not in achieving a particular state of mind, but in resting in the stillness within. Whether you practice Yoga Nidra for stress reduction, improved sleep, enhanced creativity, emotional healing, or self-discovery, may each moment of relaxation bring you closer to the peace, clarity, and inner wisdom that reside at the core of your being. As you rest in the sanctuary of deep relaxation, may you awaken to the infinite potential within and embrace the fullness of life with open arms and an open heart.

Chapter 4: Aging Gracefully: Yoga for Joint Health and Mobility

As we age, maintaining joint health and mobility becomes increasingly important for preserving our overall well-being and quality of life. Yoga offers a gentle and effective approach to supporting joint health, enhancing flexibility, and promoting mobility, enabling us to age gracefully and thrive at every stage of life. In this chapter, we will explore the role of yoga in promoting joint health and mobility, offering practices and techniques specifically designed to support the health and function of our joints as we age.

Understanding Joint Health and Mobility

Joints are the connections between bones that allow for movement and flexibility in the body. As we age, joints may become stiff, achy, or prone to injury due to factors such as decreased synovial fluid production, cartilage degeneration, and loss of muscle mass. However, with regular yoga practice, we can help to maintain and even improve joint health by lubricating the joints, strengthening the surrounding muscles, and increasing the range of motion.

The Benefits of Yoga for Joint Health and Mobility

Yoga offers a holistic approach to supporting joint health and mobility, addressing both the physical and energetic aspects of movement. Some key benefits of yoga for joint health and mobility include:

- **Improved Flexibility**: Yoga poses gently stretch and lengthen the muscles surrounding the joints, increasing flexibility and range of motion.
- **Increased Strength**: Yoga builds strength in the muscles that support and stabilize the joints, reducing the risk of injury and improving overall joint function.
- **Enhanced Circulation**: Yoga practices such as dynamic movement and breathwork promote circulation, delivering oxygen and nutrients to the joints and flushing out toxins.
- **Mind-Body Connection**: Yoga cultivates mindfulness and body awareness, allowing us to tune into the sensations and signals of our joints and move with greater ease and precision.
- **Stress Reduction**: Yoga practices such as meditation and relaxation techniques help to reduce stress and tension in the body, relieving strain on the joints and promoting relaxation.

Yoga Practices for Joint Health and Mobility

Incorporating a variety of yoga practices into your routine can help to support joint health and mobility as you age. Some key practices to consider include:

- **Gentle Yoga Poses**: Gentle yoga poses such as Cat-Cow, Child's Pose, and Gentle Twists help to lubricate the joints, release tension, and improve flexibility without putting undue stress on the body.
- **Joint-Specific Exercises**: Targeted exercises that focus on specific joints, such as wrist circles, ankle rotations, and shoulder rolls, can help to increase mobility and reduce stiffness in those areas.

- **Strength-Building Poses**: Strength-building yoga poses such as Warrior poses, Chair Pose, and Bridge Pose help to strengthen the muscles surrounding the joints, providing stability and support for healthy movement.
- **Balancing Poses**: Balancing poses such as Tree Pose, Eagle Pose, and Half Moon Pose challenge stability and proprioception, improving joint proprioception and reducing the risk of falls.
- **Breathwork and Relaxation**: Practices such as deep breathing, guided relaxation, and Yoga Nidra promote relaxation and reduce stress, relieving tension in the body and supporting overall joint health.

As we age, maintaining joint health and mobility is essential for staying active, independent, and vibrant. By incorporating yoga practices into our daily routine, we can support the health and function of our joints, enhance flexibility and range of motion, and cultivate a deep sense of vitality and well-being. Whether you're new to yoga or a seasoned practitioner, there are practices and techniques to suit everybody and every stage of life. As you embark on your journey towards aging gracefully, may you move with grace, strength, and joy, embracing the gift of movement and vitality that yoga offers at every age.

4.1 Understanding Joint Health and Common Age-Related Issues

As we age, maintaining optimal joint health becomes increasingly important for preserving mobility, flexibility, and overall quality of life. Joints are crucial for movement, providing the connections between bones that allow us to bend, twist, and move freely. However, with age, joints may experience wear and tear, leading to common age-related issues that can impact daily functioning and well-being. In this section, we will explore the anatomy of joints, common age-related issues, and how yoga can support joint health as we age.

Anatomy of Joints

Joints are complex structures made up of bones, cartilage, ligaments, tendons, and synovial fluid. The three main types of joints in the body are:

- **Synovial Joints**: These are the most common type of joint and are found in the knees, hips, shoulders, and elbows. They are surrounded by a capsule filled with synovial fluid, which lubricates the joint and reduces friction during movement.
- **Cartilaginous Joints**: These joints are made up of cartilage and are found in the spine and between the ribs and sternum. They provide stability and allow for slight movement.
- **Fibrous Joints**: These joints are connected by fibrous tissue and are found in the skull and pelvis. They provide stability and support, with little to no movement.

Common Age-Related Joint Issues

As we age, several factors can contribute to changes in joint health and function. Some common age-related joint issues include:

- **Osteoarthritis**: This is the most common form of arthritis and occurs when the cartilage that cushions the ends of bones wears down over time. It can cause pain, stiffness, and decreased range of motion in the affected joints.
- **Rheumatoid Arthritis**: This is an autoimmune condition that causes inflammation in the joints, leading to pain, swelling, and deformity. It can affect multiple joints throughout the body and can significantly impact mobility and quality of life.
- **Joint Stiffness**: As we age, joints may become stiff and less flexible due to a decrease in synovial fluid production and changes in cartilage and ligaments. This can make movement more challenging and increase the risk of injury.
- **Osteoporosis**: This is a condition characterized by a loss of bone density, which can weaken the bones and increase the risk of fractures, particularly in the spine, hips, and wrists.
- **Degenerative Disc Disease**: This is a common age-related condition that affects the intervertebral discs in the spine, leading to pain, stiffness, and decreased mobility.

How Yoga Supports Joint Health

Yoga offers a gentle and effective approach to supporting joint health as we age. Through a combination of mindful movement, stretching, strengthening, and relaxation techniques, yoga can help to:

- **Improve Flexibility**: Yoga poses gently stretch and lengthen the muscles surrounding the joints, increasing flexibility and range of motion.

- **Strengthen Muscles**: Yoga builds strength in the muscles that support and stabilize the joints, reducing the risk of injury and improving overall joint function.
- **Promote Circulation**: Yoga practices such as dynamic movement and breathwork promote circulation, delivering oxygen and nutrients to the joints and flushing out toxins.
- **Reduce Stress**: Yoga practices such as meditation and relaxation techniques help to reduce stress and tension in the body, relieving strain on the joints and promoting relaxation.
- **Enhance Mind-Body Awareness**: Yoga cultivates mindfulness and body awareness, allowing us to tune into the sensations and signals of our joints and move with greater ease and precision.

Understanding the anatomy of joints and common age-related issues is essential for maintaining optimal joint health as we age. By incorporating yoga into our daily routine, we can support joint health, enhance flexibility and mobility, and cultivate a deep sense of well-being and vitality. Whether you're new to yoga or a seasoned practitioner, there are practices and techniques to suit everybody and every stage of life. As you embark on your journey towards aging gracefully, may you move with grace, strength, and joy, embracing the gift of movement and vitality that yoga offers at every age.

4.2 Yoga Poses to Maintain Joint Flexibility

Maintaining joint flexibility is crucial for preserving mobility, preventing injury, and promoting overall well-being, especially as we age. Yoga offers a gentle and effective way to keep joints supple and mobile through a variety of poses that stretch and strengthen the muscles surrounding the joints. In this section, we will explore some key yoga poses specifically designed to maintain joint flexibility and promote joint health at every stage of life.

1. Downward-Facing Dog (Adho Mukha Svanasana)

Benefits: Downward-Facing Dog is a full-body stretch that targets the shoulders, hamstrings, calves, and ankles. It promotes flexibility in the spine, shoulders, and hips, while also strengthening the arms and legs.

How to Practice:

- Begin on your hands and knees, with your wrists aligned under your shoulders and your knees under your hips.
- Press into your palms and lift your hips up and back, coming into an inverted V shape.
- Keep your hands shoulder-width apart and your feet hip-width apart, with your heels reaching towards the ground.
- Lengthen your spine and draw your shoulder blades down your back, pressing your chest towards your thighs.
- Hold the pose for 5-10 breaths, focusing on lengthening and stretching through the entire body.

2. Extended Triangle Pose (Utthita Trikonasana)

Benefits: Extended Triangle Pose stretches the hamstrings, hips, groins, spine, and shoulders. It improves flexibility in the hips and spine, while also strengthening the legs, core, and back muscles.

How to Practice:

- Begin in a standing position with your feet about 3-4 feet apart, with your right foot turned out and your left foot turned slightly inward.
- Extend your arms out to the sides at shoulder height, parallel to the floor.
- Hinge at your right hip and reach your right hand towards your right ankle, shin, or a block placed on the floor.
- Extend your left arm up towards the ceiling, stacking your shoulders and opening your chest towards the sky.
- Keep both legs straight and engage your quadriceps, pressing into the outer edge of your left foot.
- Hold the pose for 5-10 breaths, then switch sides and repeat on the other side.

3. Seated Forward Bend (Paschimottanasana)

Benefits: Seated Forward Bend stretches the entire back side of the body, including the spine, hamstrings, and calves. It improves flexibility in the spine and hamstrings, while also calming the mind and relieving stress.

How to Practice:

- Sit on the floor with your legs extended in front of you and your feet flexed towards you.

- Inhale to lengthen your spine, then exhale to hinge at your hips and fold forward from your waist.
- Reach your hands towards your feet, ankles, or shins, keeping your spine long and your chest open.
- Relax your neck and shoulders, allowing your head to hang heavy towards your legs.
- Hold the pose for 5-10 breaths, breathing deeply into the stretch and surrendering to the release.

4. Cat-Cow Pose (Marjaryasana-Bitilasana)

Benefits: Cat-Cow Pose is a gentle, flowing movement that stretches and mobilizes the spine. It improves flexibility and mobility in the spine, shoulders, and hips, while also engaging the core muscles.

How to Practice:

- Begin on your hands and knees, with your wrists aligned under your shoulders and your knees under your hips.
- Inhale as you arch your back and lift your chest towards the ceiling, coming into Cow Pose.
- Exhale as you round your spine and tuck your chin towards your chest, coming into Cat Pose.
- Continue to flow between Cat and Cow Pose, moving with your breath and allowing your movements to be fluid and intuitive.
- Repeat for 5-10 rounds, focusing on the sensations in your spine and allowing the movement to be smooth and controlled.

5. Garland Pose (Malasana)

Benefits: Garland Pose stretches the ankles, knees, hips, and spine, while also strengthening the legs and opening the hips. It improves flexibility and mobility in the lower body, while also promoting grounding and stability.

How to Practice:

- Begin standing with your feet slightly wider than hip-width apart, with your toes turned slightly outward.
- Bend your knees and lower your hips towards the ground, coming into a deep squat position.
- Bring your palms together at your heart center, pressing your elbows into your inner thighs to open your hips.
- Lengthen your spine and lift your chest towards the sky, keeping your gaze forward.
- Hold the pose for 5-10 breaths, breathing deeply into the stretch and surrendering to the opening in your hips and groin.

Incorporating these yoga poses into your regular practice can help to maintain joint flexibility, prevent stiffness, and promote overall joint health as you age. Remember to move mindfully and honor your body's limitations, listening to your body and practicing with awareness and compassion. By prioritizing joint flexibility and mobility through yoga, you can continue to move with grace, ease, and vitality at every stage of life.

4.3 Modifications for Specific Needs and Conditions

Yoga is a practice that can be adapted to suit individuals of all ages, abilities, and physical conditions. Whether you're managing a specific health condition, injury, or limitation, there are modifications and variations of yoga poses that can help you safely and effectively reap the benefits of yoga practice. In this section, we will explore some common modifications for specific needs and conditions, empowering you to tailor your yoga practice to meet your unique needs and goals.

1. Joint Pain or Arthritis

If you experience joint pain or arthritis, it's important to practice yoga with caution and listen to your body. Here are some modifications to consider:

- **Use Props**: Use props such as blocks, bolsters, or blankets to support your body and reduce strain on your joints. For example, you can place a block under your hand in poses like Triangle Pose to reduce the distance to the floor.
- **Reduce Range of Motion**: Modify poses to reduce the range of motion in the affected joints. For example, in Warrior II Pose, you can shorten your stance and bend your front knee less deeply to reduce strain on the knees.
- **Avoid Weight-Bearing Poses**: If certain joints are particularly sensitive, avoid weight-bearing poses that put pressure on those joints. Instead, focus on seated or reclined poses that support the body and reduce strain.

2. Back Pain or Injury

Back pain or injury can make certain yoga poses challenging, but with the right modifications, you can still enjoy the benefits of yoga practice. Here are some modifications to consider:

- **Focus on Alignment**: Pay close attention to your alignment in each pose, ensuring that your spine remains in a neutral position and avoiding excessive rounding or arching of the back.
- **Use Props**: Props such as blocks, straps, or bolsters can provide support and assistance in poses that put a strain on the back. For example, you can use a bolster under your knees in Savasana to support the lower back.
- **Modify Forward Bends**: If forward bends aggravate your back pain, try bending your knees generously or practicing seated forward bends instead of standing ones. You can also use a chair for support in poses like Forward Fold.

3. Pregnancy

Pregnancy brings unique changes to the body, and it's essential to modify your yoga practice to accommodate these changes and ensure the safety of both you and your baby. Here are some modifications to consider:

- **Avoid Supine Poses**: After the first trimester, it's best to avoid lying flat on your back for extended periods, as this can compress

the vena cava and restrict blood flow to the uterus. Instead,
practice poses in a reclined or seated position.

- **Avoid Deep Twists**: Deep twists can compress the abdomen and
  may be uncomfortable during pregnancy. Instead, focus on gentle,
  open twists that allow space for your growing belly.
- **Listen to Your Body**: Pay close attention to how your body feels
  during practice, and modify or skip any poses that feel
  uncomfortable or strained. Honor your body's changing needs and
  practice with awareness and compassion.

4. High Blood Pressure or Heart Conditions

If you have high blood pressure or a heart condition, it's important to
practice yoga mindfully and avoid poses that may elevate your heart rate
or blood pressure excessively. Here are some modifications to consider:

- **Practice Gentle Poses**: Choose gentle, restorative poses that
  promote relaxation and calmness, such as Child's Pose, Legs-Up-
  the-Wall Pose, or Supported Bridge Pose.
- **Avoid Inversions**: Inversions such as Headstand or Shoulderstand
  can increase blood pressure and may not be suitable for individuals
  with high blood pressure or heart conditions. Instead, practice
  gentle forward bends and seated poses that promote grounding and
  stability.
- **Focus on Breath Awareness**: Incorporate breath awareness and
  relaxation techniques into your practice to help regulate your
  nervous system and promote overall well-being.

Yoga is a practice of self-awareness and self-care, and it's essential to honor your body's needs and limitations as you practice. By making appropriate modifications and adjustments, you can ensure that your yoga practice remains safe, effective, and enjoyable, regardless of your specific needs or conditions. Remember to listen to your body, communicate openly with your yoga teacher about any concerns or limitations, and practice with compassion and mindfulness. With the right modifications, yoga can be a valuable tool for enhancing your physical, mental, and emotional well-being, empowering you to live your best life with vitality and grace.

Chapter 5: Cultivating a Healthy Lifestyle: Integrating Yoga into Daily Routine

Incorporating yoga into your daily routine can be a transformative step towards cultivating a healthy lifestyle that nourishes your body, mind, and spirit. Yoga offers a holistic approach to well-being, providing a balance of physical movement, breathwork, mindfulness, and relaxation techniques that support overall health and vitality. In this chapter, we will explore the benefits of integrating yoga into your daily routine and offer practical tips for creating a sustainable yoga practice that enhances your quality of life.

Understanding the Benefits of Yoga

Yoga offers a multitude of benefits for physical, mental, and emotional health, making it an ideal addition to your daily routine. Some key benefits of yoga include:

- **Improved Flexibility and Strength**: Regular yoga practice helps to increase flexibility, strength, and range of motion in the body, enhancing physical fitness and reducing the risk of injury.
- **Stress Reduction**: Yoga practices such as deep breathing, meditation, and relaxation techniques help to reduce stress levels, promote relaxation, and improve overall mental well-being.
- **Enhanced Mind-Body Connection**: Yoga cultivates mindfulness and body awareness, allowing you to tune into the present moment and connect more deeply with your body, breath, and inner self.

- **Increased Energy and Vitality**: Yoga practices such as dynamic movement and breathwork help to increase energy levels, improve circulation, and promote a sense of vitality and well-being.
- **Better Sleep**: Regular yoga practice has been shown to improve sleep quality and duration, helping you to feel more rested and rejuvenated upon waking.

Tips for Integrating Yoga into Your Daily Routine

Integrating yoga into your daily routine doesn't have to be complicated or time-consuming. With a few simple adjustments, you can create space for yoga practice amidst the demands of daily life. Here are some practical tips for incorporating yoga into your daily routine:

- **Set Realistic Goals**: Start small and set realistic goals for your yoga practice. Whether it's five minutes of gentle stretching in the morning or a full-length yoga class in the evening, find a routine that works for you and commit to it consistently.
- **Create a Dedicated Space**: Designate a space in your home where you can practice yoga comfortably and without distractions. It doesn't need to be large or elaborate—simply clear a corner of a room, roll out a yoga mat and adorn the space with a few candles, cushions, or inspiring objects.
- **Schedule Regular Practice Times**: Choose specific times of day to practice yoga that align with your schedule and energy levels. Whether it's first thing in the morning to set the tone for the day or in the evening to unwind and relax before bed, find times that work best for you and stick to them consistently.

- **Mix It Up**: Keep your yoga practice fresh and engaging by exploring different styles, teachers, and lengths of practice. Try a variety of yoga classes, from gentle restorative yoga to dynamic vinyasa flow, and incorporate elements of breathwork, meditation, and mindfulness into your routine.
- **Listen to Your Body**: Honor your body's needs and limitations as you practice yoga, and modify poses or practices as necessary to suit your individual needs. Pay attention to how you feel during and after practice, and adjust your routine accordingly to support your overall well-being.

Integrating yoga into your daily routine is not just about physical exercise—it's about embracing yoga as a way of life that nurtures and supports your holistic well-being. By incorporating yoga into your daily routine, you can cultivate a healthy lifestyle that promotes physical fitness, mental clarity, emotional balance, and spiritual growth. Whether you practice for five minutes or an hour each day, the key is to approach your practice with intention, mindfulness, and dedication. As you commit to integrating yoga into your daily routine, may you discover the transformative power of yoga to enrich every aspect of your life, fostering health, happiness, and vitality for years to come.

5.1 Creating a Balanced Yoga Practice Schedule

Creating a balanced yoga practice schedule is essential for maximizing the benefits of your practice while ensuring that you address the diverse needs of your body, mind, and spirit. A well-rounded yoga practice incorporates a variety of elements, including physical movement, breathwork, meditation, and relaxation techniques, to promote overall health and well-being. In this section, we will explore how to create a balanced yoga practice schedule that meets your individual needs and supports your journey toward optimal health and vitality.

Understanding the Components of a Balanced Yoga Practice

A balanced yoga practice typically includes the following components:

- **Asana (Physical Postures)**: Asanas help to improve flexibility, strength, and balance in the body. They also promote physical fitness and reduce the risk of injury.
- **Pranayama (Breathwork)**: Pranayama techniques involve conscious control and regulation of the breath. They help to calm the mind, increase energy levels, and promote relaxation.
- **Meditation**: Meditation cultivates mindfulness and inner awareness, helping to reduce stress, improve concentration, and enhance overall mental well-being.
- **Relaxation**: Relaxation techniques such as Yoga Nidra or Savasana promote deep relaxation and rejuvenation of the body and mind.

Creating Your Yoga Practice Schedule

When creating your yoga practice schedule, consider incorporating each of these components to create a well-rounded and balanced practice. Here's how you can structure your practice schedule:

- **Daily Asana Practice**: Dedicate time each day to physical asana practice. This can range from 15 minutes to an hour, depending on your schedule and preferences. Include a mix of standing poses, seated poses, twists, backbends, forward bends, and inversions to work all areas of the body.
- **Weekly Pranayama Practice**: Set aside time each week for pranayama practice. Start with simple techniques such as deep belly breathing or alternate nostril breathing, and gradually incorporate more advanced practices as you become more comfortable.
- **Regular Meditation Sessions**: Schedule regular meditation sessions throughout the week. This can be as short as five minutes or as long as 30 minutes, depending on your availability and experience level. Choose a quiet, comfortable space where you can sit comfortably and without distractions.
- **Daily Relaxation Practice**: End each yoga session with a period of relaxation. This can include Savasana (Corpse Pose), Yoga Nidra, or a guided relaxation meditation. Allow yourself to fully relax and let go of any tension or stress in the body and mind.

Flexibility and Adaptability

Remember that your yoga practice schedule should be flexible and adaptable to accommodate changes in your schedule, energy levels, and needs. If you're short on time one day, focus on a shorter, more condensed practice. If you're feeling tired or stressed, prioritize relaxation techniques and gentle, restorative poses. Listen to your body and honor its needs, adjusting your practice schedule accordingly.

By creating a balanced yoga practice schedule that incorporates a variety of elements, you can cultivate health, vitality, and well-being in all areas of your life. Whether you practice for a few minutes or an hour each day, the key is to approach your practice with intention, mindfulness, and dedication. As you commit to creating a balanced yoga practice schedule, may you discover the transformative power of yoga to nourish your body, calm your mind, and uplift your spirit, fostering health, happiness, and harmony in your life.

5.2 Incorporating Yoga into Exercise Regimens

Integrating yoga into your exercise regimen can be a valuable addition to your fitness routine, enhancing the benefits of your workouts and promoting overall health and well-being. Yoga offers a unique combination of physical movement, breathwork, and mindfulness practices that complement a wide range of exercises, from cardio and strength training to endurance and flexibility training. In this section, we will explore how to incorporate yoga into your exercise regimen to maximize the benefits of both practices and create a balanced and holistic approach to fitness.

Understanding the Benefits of Combining Yoga with Other Exercises

Combining yoga with other forms of exercise offers a multitude of benefits for physical, mental, and emotional health:

- **Improved Flexibility**: Yoga helps to increase flexibility and range of motion in the body, enhancing performance and reducing the risk of injury during other forms of exercise.

- **Enhanced Strength**: Yoga builds strength in both large and small muscle groups, improving stability, balance, and overall muscle tone.
- **Better Alignment and Posture**: Yoga promotes proper alignment and posture, helping to prevent muscle imbalances and alleviate strain on the joints during other forms of exercise.
- **Increased Mind-Body Awareness**: Yoga cultivates mindfulness and body awareness, allowing you to tune into the sensations and signals of your body during other exercises, leading to more efficient and effective workouts.
- **Reduced Stress and Recovery**: Yoga practices such as deep breathing and relaxation techniques help to reduce stress levels and promote recovery and rejuvenation after intense workouts.

Tips for Incorporating Yoga into Your Exercise Regimen

Here are some practical tips for incorporating yoga into your exercise regimen:

- **Pre-Workout Warm-Up**: Start your workout with a brief yoga warm-up to prepare your body for exercise. Include dynamic stretches, gentle movement, and breathwork to loosen up tight muscles and joints and increase blood flow to the muscles.
- **Post-Workout Stretching**: End your workout with a yoga cool-down to stretch and lengthen the muscles worked during exercise. Focus on poses that target the areas of the body that were most engaged during your workout, such as hip openers after running or shoulder stretches after strength training.

- **Cross-Training with Yoga**: Incorporate yoga into your weekly exercise routine as a form of cross-training. Balance high-intensity workouts with gentler, more restorative yoga practices to prevent burnout and promote recovery.
- **Yoga for Active Recovery**: On rest days or recovery days, engage in gentle yoga practices to promote relaxation, release tension, and support the body's natural healing process. Choose restorative yoga poses and relaxation techniques to soothe tired muscles and calm the mind.
- **Mindful Movement**: Approach your yoga practice with mindfulness and intention, focusing on the quality of movement and breath rather than intensity or achievement. Listen to your body and honor its needs, modifying poses as necessary to suit your capabilities and limitations.

By incorporating yoga into your exercise regimen, you can enhance the benefits of your workouts and create a balanced and holistic approach to fitness. Whether you practice yoga as a warm-up, cool-down, cross-training activity, or active recovery tool, the key is to approach your practice with mindfulness, intention, and dedication. As you combine yoga with other forms of exercise, may you discover the transformative power of movement, breath, and mindfulness to nourish your body, calm your mind, and uplift your spirit, fostering health, happiness, and vitality in every aspect of your life.

5.3 Nutrition Tips for Supporting Youthful Vitality

Maintaining youthful vitality involves more than just physical exercise and mental well-being—it also depends on proper nutrition to fuel your body and support overall health and vitality. A balanced and nutrient-rich diet plays a crucial role in promoting longevity, energy, and vitality, helping you look and feel your best at every age. In this section, we will explore nutrition tips for supporting youthful vitality and incorporating healthy eating habits into your lifestyle.

Eat a Variety of Nutrient-Rich Foods

- **Colorful Fruits and Vegetables**: Incorporate a variety of colorful fruits and vegetables into your meals to provide essential vitamins, minerals, and antioxidants that support overall health and vitality.
- **Lean Protein Sources**: Include lean protein sources such as poultry, fish, tofu, legumes, and nuts in your diet to support muscle growth and repair, promote satiety, and maintain energy levels.
- **Healthy Fats**: Choose healthy fats from sources such as avocados, nuts, seeds, and olive oil to support brain health, reduce inflammation, and promote heart health.
- **Whole Grains**: Opt for whole grains such as quinoa, brown rice, oats, and whole wheat bread to provide fiber, vitamins, and minerals that support digestion and energy production.

Hydrate Your Body

- **Drink Plenty of Water**: Stay hydrated by drinking plenty of water throughout the day. Aim for at least eight glasses of water daily, and adjust your intake based on activity level, climate, and individual needs.
- **Limit Sugary Beverages**: Avoid sugary drinks such as soda, fruit juice, and energy drinks, which can contribute to dehydration, blood sugar spikes, and energy crashes.
- **Herbal Teas**: Enjoy herbal teas such as green tea, chamomile, or ginger tea as a hydrating and refreshing alternative to sugary beverages.

Prioritize Whole, Unprocessed Foods

- **Minimize Processed Foods**: Limit your intake of processed and packaged foods high in added sugars, unhealthy fats, and artificial ingredients. Instead, focus on whole, unprocessed foods that nourish your body and support optimal health.
- **Cook at Home**: Prepare meals at home using fresh, whole ingredients whenever possible. Cooking at home allows you to control the quality and quantity of ingredients, making it easier to make nutritious choices.
- **Read Labels**: When purchasing packaged foods, read labels carefully and choose options with minimal ingredients and no added sugars or artificial additives.

Practice Mindful Eating

- **Eat Mindfully**: Practice mindful eating by paying attention to your body's hunger and fullness cues, eating slowly, and savoring each bite. This helps prevent overeating and promotes greater satisfaction with your meals.
- **Listen to Your Body**: Tune into your body's signals of hunger, thirst, and satisfaction, and honor its needs without judgment or restriction.
- **Practice Gratitude**: Cultivate gratitude for the nourishing foods that fuel your body and support your health and vitality. Approach eating with a sense of appreciation and enjoyment, savoring the flavors and textures of your meals.

By prioritizing nutrient-rich foods, staying hydrated, and practicing mindful eating, you can support youthful vitality and overall well-being at every age. Incorporate these nutrition tips into your lifestyle to fuel your body with the nourishment it needs to thrive, look radiant, and feel vibrant. Remember that healthy eating is not about perfection—it's about making sustainable choices that support your health and vitality for the long term. As you nourish your body, may you also nourish your life, embracing the joy, energy, and vitality that come from living in alignment with your healthiest self.

Chapter 6: Overcoming Challenges: Addressing Obstacles to Practice

Embarking on a journey of yoga practice is a rewarding endeavor, but it can also come with its fair share of challenges and obstacles along the way. From lack of time and motivation to physical limitations and self-doubt, many factors can hinder our commitment to regular practice. In this chapter, we will explore common challenges faced by practitioners and offer strategies for overcoming these obstacles to cultivate a sustainable and fulfilling yoga practice.

Identifying Common Challenges

- **Time Constraints**: Busy schedules and hectic lifestyles often leave little time for self-care and exercise, making it challenging to prioritize yoga practice amidst competing demands.
- **Lack of Motivation**: Finding the motivation to roll out the yoga mat and practice can be difficult, especially on days when you're feeling tired, stressed, or unmotivated.
- **Physical Limitations**: Physical injuries, chronic conditions, or mobility issues can present barriers to certain yoga poses or practices, leading to frustration and discouragement.
- **Self-Doubt and Perfectionism**: Negative self-talk and feelings of inadequacy can undermine confidence and enjoyment in yoga practice, leading to self-imposed pressure to perform perfectly.

Strategies for Overcoming Obstacles

- **Set Realistic Goals**: Break down your yoga practice goals into manageable and realistic steps. Start with small, achievable goals that align with your schedule and capabilities, and gradually build upon them over time.
- **Prioritize Self-Care**: Recognize the importance of self-care and prioritize time for yoga practice as an essential component of your overall well-being. Treat your yoga practice as a non-negotiable commitment to yourself, just like eating, sleeping, or brushing your teeth.
- **Create a Consistent Routine**: Establish a routine for your yoga practice by scheduling specific times for practice each day or week. Consistency is key to building a sustainable practice and overcoming resistance or inertia.
- **Find Accountability and Support**: Enlist the support of friends, family members, or a yoga buddy to hold you accountable and provide encouragement on your yoga journey. Joining a yoga class or community can also offer a sense of camaraderie and motivation to stay committed to your practice.
- **Practice Self-Compassion**: Be kind and compassionate towards yourself, especially when facing challenges or setbacks in your yoga practice. Embrace the imperfections and fluctuations of your practice with a sense of acceptance and curiosity, rather than judgment or criticism.
- **Modify and Adapt**: Honor your body's needs and limitations by modifying yoga poses or practices to suit your capabilities. Focus on what you can do rather than what you can't, and approach your practice with an attitude of curiosity and exploration.

Cultivating Resilience and Persistence

Overcoming obstacles in your yoga practice requires resilience, persistence, and a willingness to adapt and grow. Embrace challenges as opportunities for learning and growth, and trust in your ability to navigate them with grace and resilience. Remember that progress in yoga is not linear—there will be ups and downs along the way, but each obstacle you overcome strengthens your resolve and deepens your commitment to your practice.

By acknowledging and addressing the challenges that arise in your yoga practice, you can cultivate a deeper sense of resilience, commitment, and fulfillment on your journey toward health and well-being. Approach obstacles as opportunities for growth and self-discovery, and trust in your ability to overcome them with patience, perseverance, and self-compassion. As you navigate the ups and downs of your yoga practice, may you find strength, inspiration, and joy in the journey, embracing each moment with openness, curiosity, and grace.

6.1 Time Management Strategies for Busy Schedules

Managing a busy schedule can often feel like a juggling act, with competing demands pulling you in multiple directions. Finding time for yoga practice amidst work, family, and other obligations can be challenging, but with effective time management strategies, it's possible to carve out dedicated time for self-care and exercise. In this section, we will explore practical time management strategies to help you prioritize and integrate yoga practice into your busy schedule.

1. Schedule Your Practice

Block Out Time: Treat your yoga practice as a non-negotiable appointment by blocking out dedicated time for it in your calendar. Choose times of day that work best for you and align with your energy levels, whether it's early morning, during your lunch break, or in the evening.

Set Reminders: Use alarms, notifications, or reminders to prompt you to practice at your scheduled time. Set a reminder on your phone or calendar app to signal the start of your yoga session and help you stay on track.

2. Combine Activities

Multitask Mindfully: Look for opportunities to combine yoga practice with other activities in your daily routine. For example, practice mindfulness and deep breathing while commuting, incorporate standing poses or stretches while brushing your teeth or waiting in line or do gentle yoga poses while watching TV.

Family Yoga: Involve your family members in your yoga practice by incorporating family yoga sessions into your schedule. Practice simple poses together, encourage children to join in, and make it a fun and bonding experience for the whole family.

3. Short and Sweet Sessions

Embrace Micro-Practices: Break down your yoga practice into shorter, more manageable sessions that fit into your busy schedule. Even just 10-15 minutes of yoga can be beneficial and rejuvenating. Find pockets of time throughout the day to sneak in quick yoga sessions whenever possible.

Focus on Key Poses: Prioritize key yoga poses or sequences that target areas of tension or stiffness in your body. Choose poses that offer the most bang for your buck in terms of stretching, strengthening, and relaxation, such as Sun Salutations, forward bends, and gentle twists.

4. Create a Dedicated Space

Designate a Yoga Corner: Set up a dedicated space in your home where you can practice yoga comfortably and without distractions. Create a peaceful and inviting atmosphere with a yoga mat, cushions, candles, and any other props or accessories that inspire you to practice.

Keep it Simple: Your yoga space doesn't need to be large or elaborate—just a quiet corner or area free from clutter and distractions will suffice. Make it a sacred space where you can retreat to reconnect with yourself and your practice.

5. Prioritize Self-Care

Make Yourself a Priority: Recognize the importance of self-care and prioritize time for yoga practice as an essential component of your overall well-being. Remember that taking care of yourself allows you to show up as your best self in other areas of your life.

Set Boundaries: Learn to say no to non-essential commitments and obligations that detract from your well-being and prevent you from prioritizing self-care. Establish healthy boundaries around your time and energy, and allocate time for yoga practice as a non-negotiable part of your routine.

By implementing these time management strategies, you can find balance amidst busyness and prioritize yoga practice as an integral part of your daily routine. Remember that consistency is key, and even small, incremental steps toward your yoga goals can lead to significant progress over time. By making self-care a priority and carving out dedicated time for yoga practice, you can reap the countless benefits of this ancient practice and cultivate health, vitality, and well-being in your life.

6.2 Dealing with Physical Limitations and Injuries

Physical limitations and injuries can present significant challenges to your yoga practice, but with the right approach and mindset, it's possible to adapt and modify your practice to accommodate your unique needs. Whether you're recovering from an injury, managing a chronic condition, or experiencing mobility limitations, some strategies and modifications can help you continue to benefit from yoga practice while minimizing the risk of further injury or discomfort. In this section, we will explore how to deal with physical limitations and injuries in your yoga practice with sensitivity, awareness, and self-care.

1. Listen to Your Body

Practice Mindful Awareness: Tune into your body's signals and sensations during yoga practice, paying attention to areas of discomfort, tension, or pain. Practice mindfulness and body awareness to discern between sensations that indicate progress and those that signal potential injury.

Honor Your Limits: Respect your body's limitations and avoid pushing yourself beyond your comfort zone or into pain. Embrace the concept of Ahimsa, or non-harming, by practicing with compassion and kindness towards yourself.

2. Communicate with Your Instructor

Open Communication: Communicate openly and honestly with your yoga instructor about any physical limitations, injuries, or concerns you may have. Your instructor can offer guidance, modifications, and support to help you practice safely and effectively.

Ask for Modifications: Don't hesitate to ask for modifications or alternatives to traditional yoga poses that may exacerbate your condition or discomfort. Your instructor can suggest variations that accommodate your needs and support your healing process.

3. Modify and Adapt Poses

Use Props: Props such as blocks, straps, bolsters, and blankets can provide support and assistance in yoga poses, making them more accessible and comfortable. Experiment with different props to find variations that alleviate strain on your body.

Focus on Alignment: Pay close attention to proper alignment in each pose, ensuring that your body is supported and stable. Modify poses as needed to maintain alignment and avoid putting excessive stress on vulnerable areas.

4. Explore Gentle and Restorative Practices

Choose Gentle Styles: Explore gentle styles of yoga such as Hatha, Yin, or Restorative yoga, which emphasize slow, mindful movement and longer holds in supported poses. These styles are gentle on the body and can be particularly beneficial for individuals with physical limitations or injuries.

Practice Yoga Nidra: Incorporate Yoga Nidra, or guided relaxation meditation, into your practice to promote deep relaxation and healing at both the physical and emotional levels. Yoga Nidra can be practiced lying down and requires minimal physical exertion.

5. Work with a Physical Therapist

Seek Professional Guidance: Consider working with a physical therapist or healthcare provider who specializes in rehabilitative therapy or sports medicine. A qualified professional can assess your condition, provide personalized recommendations, and design a tailored exercise program to support your recovery and well-being.

Integrate Therapy Techniques: Integrate therapeutic techniques recommended by your physical therapist, such as gentle stretches, strengthening exercises, and mobility drills, into your yoga practice to support healing and rehabilitation.

By practicing with awareness, adaptability, and self-compassion, you can navigate physical limitations and injuries in your yoga practice with grace and resilience. Remember that yoga is a personal journey, and there is no one-size-fits-all approach. Listen to your body, communicate openly with your instructor, and explore modifications and variations that support your healing process and promote overall well-being. With patience, persistence, and a commitment to self-care, you can continue to experience the transformative benefits of yoga practice, regardless of any physical limitations or challenges you may face.

6.3 Motivational Techniques to Stay Consistent

Staying consistent with your yoga practice can sometimes be a challenge, especially when life gets busy or motivation wanes. However, by implementing motivational techniques and strategies, you can cultivate a sense of dedication, commitment, and enthusiasm to keep showing up on the mat, day after day. In this section, we will explore effective motivational techniques to help you stay consistent with your yoga practice and maintain momentum on your journey toward health, well-being, and self-discovery.

1. Set Clear and Achievable Goals

Define Your Why: Clarify your reasons for practicing yoga and identify what you hope to achieve through your practice. Whether it's improving flexibility, reducing stress, or cultivating inner peace, having a clear sense of purpose can fuel your motivation and keep you focused on your goals.

Break it Down: Break down your goals into smaller, actionable steps that are specific, measurable, achievable, relevant, and time-bound (SMART). Celebrate each milestone along the way, no matter how small, and use your progress as motivation to keep moving forward.

2. Create a Supportive Environment

Surround Yourself with Positivity: Surround yourself with positive influences and supportive individuals who encourage and uplift you on your yoga journey. Join a yoga community, attend classes, or connect with like-minded practitioners online to share experiences, challenges, and inspiration.

Designate a Sacred Space: Create a dedicated space in your home where you can practice yoga comfortably and without distractions. Make it a sacred space that inspires and uplifts you, and return to it regularly as a sanctuary for your practice.

3. Find Joy and Inspiration

Explore Different Styles: Experiment with different styles of yoga to find what resonates with you and brings you joy. Whether it's a dynamic vinyasa flow, gentle restorative yoga, or meditative yin yoga, choose practices that nourish your body, mind, and spirit.

Seek Inspiration: Draw inspiration from yoga teachers, books, podcasts, videos, or social media channels that inspire and motivate you. Find role models who embody the qualities and values you admire, and let their wisdom and guidance fuel your practice.

4. Practice Self-Compassion and Acceptance

Embrace Imperfection: Let go of perfectionism and embrace the imperfections and fluctuations of your practice with self-compassion and acceptance. Remember that progress in yoga is not linear, and every practice is an opportunity for growth and learning.

Be Kind to Yourself: Treat yourself with kindness, patience, and understanding, especially on days when you're feeling tired, unmotivated, or discouraged. Celebrate your efforts and accomplishments, no matter how small, and cultivate a sense of gratitude for the gift of yoga in your life.

5. Stay Consistent with Routine and Ritual

Establish Rituals: Create rituals and routines around your yoga practice to anchor it firmly into your daily life. Whether it's practicing at the same time each day, lighting a candle, or incorporating breathwork or meditation, establish habits that signal to your brain that it's time for practice.

Start Small: If consistency feels overwhelming, start with small, manageable commitments that are easy to maintain. Even just a few minutes of yoga each day can make a significant difference over time, and consistency is more important than duration.

By incorporating these motivational techniques into your yoga practice, you can cultivate a growth mindset, resilience, and dedication to stay consistent on your journey of self-discovery and well-being. Remember that motivation may ebb and flow, but by nurturing your practice with intention, joy, and self-compassion, you can create a sustainable and fulfilling yoga journey that enriches every aspect of your life. As you continue to show up on the mat, may you find inspiration, empowerment, and transformation in the practice of yoga, fostering health, happiness, and vitality for years to come.

Chapter 7: Beyond the Mat: Yoga's Impact on Relationships and Community

Yoga is not just a solitary practice confined to the mat—it has the power to transcend individual boundaries and deeply impact relationships and communities. Beyond the physical postures and breathwork, yoga fosters connections, empathy, and compassion, both with ourselves and with others. In this chapter, we will explore the profound impact of yoga on relationships and community, highlighting its ability to cultivate deeper connections, foster social support, and inspire collective transformation.

1. Cultivating Connection and Empathy

Self-Reflection: Yoga encourages self-reflection and introspection, fostering a deeper understanding and acceptance of oneself. By cultivating self-awareness and compassion on the mat, practitioners develop greater empathy and understanding towards others in their lives.

Compassionate Communication: Yoga teaches mindful communication and active listening, enabling practitioners to communicate more effectively and empathetically in their relationships. By honing these skills, individuals can navigate conflicts with greater sensitivity and understanding, fostering deeper connections and mutual respect.

2. Fostering Social Support and Community

Yoga Sangha: The concept of Sangha, or spiritual community, is central to yoga philosophy. Yoga classes and communities provide a supportive environment where practitioners can come together to share experiences, challenges, and insights, fostering a sense of belonging and connection.

Shared Values: Yoga communities often share common values such as kindness, compassion, and mindfulness, creating a supportive and inclusive space for individuals from diverse backgrounds to come together in pursuit of common goals and aspirations.

3. Inspiring Collective Transformation

Seva (Selfless Service): Yoga inspires individuals to engage in Seva, or selfless service, as a means of giving back to their communities and making a positive impact in the world. Whether through volunteer work, activism, or social outreach initiatives, practitioners embody the spirit of Seva to create positive change on both personal and societal levels.

Yoga Off the Mat: The principles and teachings of yoga extend beyond the confines of the mat and into everyday life. By applying yoga philosophy and values to their interactions with others and their involvement in their communities, practitioners become agents of transformation, inspiring positive change and social justice.

Yoga's impact extends far beyond the physical postures and breathwork—it has the power to transform relationships, foster community, and inspire collective change. By cultivating connection, empathy, and compassion in our relationships and communities, we harness the transformative potential of yoga to create a more compassionate, inclusive, and interconnected world. As we continue on our yoga journey, may we embody the principles of love, kindness, and unity, and may our practice catalyze positive change in ourselves and in the world around us.

7.1 Yoga as a Tool for Cultivating Compassion and Empathy

Yoga serves as a powerful tool for cultivating compassion and empathy, both toward ourselves and towards others. Through the practice of yoga, individuals develop a deeper understanding and acceptance of themselves, which lays the foundation for extending compassion and empathy to those around them. In this section, we will explore how yoga fosters these qualities and empowers practitioners to embody compassion and empathy in their lives.

Self-Compassion on the Mat

Non-Judgmental Awareness: Yoga encourages practitioners to cultivate non-judgmental awareness of their thoughts, emotions, and physical sensations on the mat. By observing without judgment, individuals develop greater self-compassion and acceptance of themselves as they are, imperfections and all.

Gentleness and Kindness: The physical postures of yoga provide opportunities to practice gentleness and kindness towards oneself. By approaching each pose with patience, self-care, and self-compassion, practitioners learn to treat themselves with the same kindness they would extend to a dear friend.

Extending Compassion to Others

Empathy in Action: Through yoga, individuals develop a deeper sense of empathy and understanding towards others. By cultivating awareness of their struggles and vulnerabilities, practitioners are better able to empathize with the experiences and challenges of those around them, fostering deeper connections and mutual support.

Compassionate Action: Yoga inspires practitioners to translate their compassion into action, both on and off the mat. Whether through acts of kindness, service to others, or advocacy for social justice, individuals harness the transformative power of compassion to create positive change in their communities and the world.

Embracing Interconnectedness

Unity and Interconnectedness: Yoga philosophy emphasizes the interconnectedness of all beings and the underlying unity of existence. By recognizing the inherent interconnectedness of humanity, practitioners develop a sense of solidarity and compassion towards all living beings, fostering a more inclusive and compassionate society.

Seva (Selfless Service): The practice of Seva, or selfless service, is integral to yoga philosophy. By engaging in acts of service and altruism, practitioners express their compassion and empathy in tangible ways, contributing to the well-being and upliftment of others without expectation of personal gain.

Yoga serves as a transformative path for cultivating compassion and empathy in our lives. Through the practice of self-compassion, empathy towards others, and a recognition of our interconnectedness, practitioners embody the principles of love, kindness, and understanding both on and off the mat. As we continue on our yoga journey, may we cultivate compassion and empathy as guiding principles, fostering greater harmony, connection, and well-being in ourselves and in the world around us.

7.2 Partner Yoga: Strengthening Bonds through Practice

Partner yoga, also known as acro-yoga or couples yoga, offers a unique opportunity for individuals to deepen their connections with others while exploring the transformative power of yoga together. By practicing yoga in tandem with a partner, practitioners not only enhance their physical strength, flexibility, and balance but also foster trust, communication, and intimacy in their relationships. In this comprehensive guide to partner yoga, we will delve into the principles, benefits, techniques, and poses of partner yoga, highlighting its potential to strengthen bonds and cultivate harmony in relationships.

Understanding Partner Yoga

Partner yoga is a collaborative practice in which two individuals support and assist each other in performing yoga poses, often incorporating elements of balance, strength, and flexibility. Unlike traditional solo yoga practice, partner yoga emphasizes cooperation, communication, and connection between partners, creating a shared experience of movement, breath, and presence.

Benefits of Partner Yoga

- **Enhanced Communication**: Partner yoga requires clear and effective communication between partners to coordinate movements, offer support, and ensure safety. By practicing communication skills such as active listening and verbal cues, partners strengthen their ability to communicate openly and effectively in their relationship.

- **Trust and Vulnerability**: Partner yoga fosters trust and vulnerability as partners rely on each other for support, balance, and stability. By trusting their partner to hold them safely in challenging poses, individuals deepen their sense of trust and intimacy in their relationship, creating a safe space for vulnerability and exploration.
- **Physical Connection**: Partner yoga encourages physical connection and touch between partners, promoting intimacy, closeness, and affection. Through gentle touch, partners experience a deeper sense of connection and presence, fostering emotional intimacy and bonding.
- **Shared Experience**: Partner yoga creates a shared experience of movement, breath, and presence, strengthening the bond between partners and deepening their connection. By sharing the challenges and triumphs of the practice, partners cultivate a sense of camaraderie and unity, enriching their relationship.

Techniques and Practices

- **Warm-Up and Preparation**: Begin partner yoga practice with a gentle warm-up to prepare the body and mind for movement. Incorporate joint mobilization exercises, gentle stretches, and breathwork to release tension and establish a sense of connection between partners.
- **Partner-Assisted Poses**: Explore a variety of partner-assisted yoga poses that emphasize trust, communication, and cooperation. Start with foundational poses such as partner forward fold, partner

backbend, and partner twist, gradually progressing to more advanced poses as comfort and trust between partners increase.

- **Spotting and Support**: Practice spotting and supporting techniques to ensure safety and stability in partner yoga poses. Offer verbal cues, physical support, and spotting assistance as needed to help your partner maintain balance and alignment in challenging poses.
- **Breath Synchronization**: Cultivate breath synchronization between partners by coordinating inhales and exhales during movement. Encourage partners to synchronize their breath with each other, creating a harmonious flow of energy and connection between their movements.

Partner Yoga Poses

- **Partner Forward Fold**: Stand facing each other with feet hip-width apart. Hold hands and hinge forward at the hips, keeping the spine long and the knees slightly bent. Lean back and gently pull each other forward, deepening the stretch in the hamstrings and lower back.
- **Double Downward Dog**: Begin in a downward-facing dog pose with partners facing each other. Place hands on each other's lower back or hips for support. Press into the hands and feet to lengthen the spine and deepen the stretch in the shoulders and hamstrings.
- **Flying Eagle Pose**: Stand side by side with partners facing the same direction. Lift one leg and cross it over the other partner's thigh, hooking the foot behind their calf. Extend the arms out to the sides and interlace fingers, lifting the arms overhead to deepen the stretch in the shoulders and chest.

- **Seated Twist**: Sit back to back with partners, legs extended and knees bent. Inhale to lengthen the spine, and exhale to twist to one side, placing one hand on the opposite knee and the other hand on the floor behind you. Hold the twist for several breaths, then switch sides.

Safety Guidelines

- **Clear Communication**: Maintain clear and open communication with your partner throughout the practice. Use verbal cues, hand signals, or eye contact to communicate intentions, needs, and boundaries.
- **Respect Physical Limitations**: Honor your own and your partner's physical limitations and capabilities. Avoid pushing yourself or your partner into poses that feel uncomfortable or unsafe, and respect each other's boundaries at all times.
- **Use Props and Support**: Incorporate props such as blocks, blankets, or straps to provide additional support and stability in partner yoga poses. Use props mindfully to enhance comfort and safety for both partners.
- **Stay Present and Mindful**: Cultivate mindfulness and presence in partner yoga practice by staying focused on the sensations, breath, and connection between partners. Avoid distractions and maintain awareness of your body and your partner's body throughout the practice.

Partner yoga offers a unique and transformative opportunity for individuals to deepen their connections with others while exploring the transformative power of yoga together. By practicing trust, communication, and intimacy through shared movement, breath, and presence, partners cultivate stronger bonds and greater harmony in their relationships. As partners embark on their journey of partner yoga together, may they embrace the practice with openness, curiosity, and love, nurturing the connection and unity that exists between them both on and off the mat.

7.3 Building Supportive Yoga Communities: Fostering Connection, Growth, and Well-being

Yoga communities serve as nurturing environments where individuals come together to share their love for yoga, support one another on their journey of self-discovery, and cultivate a sense of belonging and connection. By fostering a supportive and inclusive community, yoga studios, teachers, and practitioners create spaces that empower individuals to explore their practice, deepen their understanding of yoga, and experience transformational growth on physical, mental, and spiritual levels. In this comprehensive guide to building supportive yoga communities, we will explore the principles, practices, benefits, and strategies for creating spaces that foster connection, growth, and well-being for all.

Understanding Supportive Yoga Communities

Supportive yoga communities are characterized by a sense of inclusivity, acceptance, and mutual support among members. These communities provide a safe and welcoming space where individuals from diverse backgrounds and experiences can come together to practice yoga, share insights and experiences, and support each other on their journey of self-discovery and personal growth.

Benefits of Supportive Yoga Communities

- **Sense of Belonging**: Supportive yoga communities offer a sense of belonging and connection for individuals who may feel isolated or disconnected in other areas of their lives. By providing a supportive and inclusive environment, these communities foster a sense of belonging and camaraderie among members.
- **Emotional Support**: Yoga communities serve as sources of emotional support and encouragement for individuals facing challenges or transitions in their lives. Through shared experiences, empathy, and compassion, community members offer support, understanding, and guidance to one another, fostering resilience and well-being.
- **Accountability and Motivation**: Supportive yoga communities provide accountability and motivation for individuals to maintain a regular yoga practice. By participating in group classes, workshops, or events, members feel motivated to show up consistently and stay committed to their practice, knowing that they are part of a supportive community that values their presence and participation.
- **Learning and Growth**: Supportive yoga communities offer opportunities for learning, growth, and self-discovery through workshops, seminars, and gatherings. By sharing knowledge, insights, and experiences, community members deepen their understanding of yoga philosophy, anatomy, and practice, enriching their journey of self-discovery and transformation.

Strategies for Building Supportive Yoga Communities

- **Create a Welcoming Environment**: Foster a welcoming and inclusive environment in your yoga studio or community space by greeting newcomers with warmth and kindness, offering assistance and guidance as needed, and creating opportunities for connection and conversation among members.
- **Cultivate Connection and Engagement**: Create opportunities for connection and engagement among community members through group classes, workshops, events, and social gatherings. Encourage members to share their experiences, insights, and challenges, fostering a sense of connection and support.
- **Facilitate Peer Support**: Facilitate peer support and mentorship programs within the community to connect individuals with similar interests, goals, or experiences. Pair experienced practitioners with newcomers or individuals facing similar challenges to provide support, guidance, and encouragement on their yoga journey.
- **Offer Diverse Programming**: Offer a diverse range of programming and classes to cater to the needs and interests of community members. Include classes for beginners, advanced practitioners, seniors, children, and individuals with specific interests or needs, ensuring that everyone feels welcomed and supported in their practice.
- **Emphasize Inclusivity and Accessibility**: Prioritize inclusivity and accessibility in your yoga community by offering classes and events that are accessible to individuals of all ages, abilities, and backgrounds. Provide accommodations and modifications as needed to ensure that everyone feels welcomed and able to participate fully in the community.
- **Encourage Collaboration and Cooperation**: Encourage collaboration and cooperation among community members by

facilitating group projects, events, or initiatives that bring individuals together to work towards a common goal or shared purpose. Foster a sense of teamwork, camaraderie, and collective responsibility within the community.

- **Celebrate Achievements and Milestones**: Celebrate achievements and milestones within the community by acknowledging and honoring the accomplishments of individual members. Recognize progress, growth, and contributions to the community, and celebrate successes together as a collective.

Building a supportive yoga community requires intentional effort, compassion, and dedication to creating spaces that foster connection, growth, and well-being for all. By prioritizing inclusivity, empathy, and collaboration, yoga communities can serve as sources of inspiration, empowerment, and transformation for individuals on their journey of self-discovery and personal growth. As we continue to cultivate supportive yoga communities, may we embrace the principles of unity, compassion, and connection, nurturing the bonds that unite us and fostering a sense of belonging and well-being for all.

Chapter 8: Aging with Grace: Wisdom from Seasoned Yogis

As we journey through life, the practice of yoga offers invaluable guidance and support for navigating the challenges and blessings of aging with grace and wisdom. In this chapter, we will explore the insights, experiences, and wisdom of seasoned yogis who have embraced yoga as a lifelong practice, discovering resilience, vitality, and inner peace as they age gracefully. Drawing upon their collective wisdom, we will uncover the transformative power of yoga in fostering physical vitality, mental clarity, and spiritual resilience as we navigate the journey of aging.

Embracing the Wisdom of Experience

Seasoned yogis offer a wealth of wisdom and insight gleaned from years of dedicated practice and lived experience. Through their commitment to yoga, these individuals have cultivated resilience, adaptability, and acceptance in the face of the inevitable changes and challenges of aging. By embracing the wisdom of experience, seasoned yogis inspire us to approach the process of aging with curiosity, gratitude, and a sense of adventure.

Cultivating Physical Vitality

Yoga serves as a powerful tool for maintaining physical vitality and well-being as we age. Through regular practice, seasoned yogis nourish and strengthen their bodies, enhancing flexibility, mobility, and strength to support active and vibrant lifestyles. By incorporating gentle movement, breathwork, and mindfulness practices into their daily routines, seasoned yogis cultivate resilience and vitality, empowering themselves to navigate the physical challenges of aging with grace and ease.

Nurturing Mental Clarity and Resilience

The practice of yoga offers profound benefits for mental clarity and emotional resilience, supporting seasoned yogis in navigating the complexities of aging with equanimity and grace. Through meditation, mindfulness, and self-reflection, seasoned yogis cultivate inner peace, wisdom, and emotional balance, fostering resilience in the face of life's inevitable ups and downs. By nurturing a mindful awareness of thoughts, emotions, and sensations, seasoned yogis cultivate a sense of clarity and presence that empowers them to approach the aging process with acceptance and serenity.

Embracing Spiritual Resilience

Yoga provides a pathway for nurturing spiritual resilience and deepening our connection to the innermost dimensions of our being as we age. Through the practice of self-inquiry, devotion, and surrender, seasoned yogis tap into a wellspring of inner wisdom, compassion, and spiritual insight that sustains them through life's transitions and challenges. By cultivating a sense of surrender and trust in the unfolding journey of life, seasoned yogis embrace the process of aging as an opportunity for spiritual growth, awakening, and transformation.

As we journey through the stages of life, the practice of yoga offers invaluable guidance and support for aging with grace, vitality, and wisdom. Drawing upon the wisdom of seasoned yogis, we discover the transformative power of yoga in fostering physical vitality, mental clarity, and spiritual resilience as we navigate the journey of aging. By embracing the practice of yoga as a lifelong journey of self-discovery and self-care, we cultivate resilience, acceptance, and gratitude for the precious gift of life in all its phases. As we honor the wisdom of our elders and embrace the teachings of yoga, may we age with grace, dignity, and a deep sense of reverence for the sacred journey of life.

8.1 Personal Stories of Transformation through Yoga

Yoga is not just a physical practice; it is a journey of self-discovery, healing, and transformation. In this chapter, we will explore the personal stories of individuals whose lives have been profoundly impacted by the practice of yoga. Through their experiences, challenges, and triumphs, we will witness the transformative power of yoga to heal the body, calm the mind, and awaken the spirit. These stories serve as testaments to the profound and lasting impact of yoga on our lives, inspiring us to embark on our journey of self-discovery and transformation through the practice of yoga.

Finding Healing and Strength: Sarah's Story

Sarah's journey with yoga began at a time of deep personal struggle and physical pain. Suffering from chronic back pain and emotional distress, Sarah felt lost and disconnected from herself and the world around her.

Desperate for relief, she turned to yoga as a last resort, hoping to find healing and strength amidst the darkness.

Through the practice of yoga, Sarah discovered a profound sense of healing and empowerment that transformed her life in ways she never imagined possible. With each breath and movement, she began to release tension and pain held within her body, cultivating a newfound sense of strength and resilience. Through mindfulness and self-compassion, she learned to navigate the ups and downs of life with grace and equanimity, embracing the present moment with an open heart and mind.

Today, Sarah's life is a testament to the transformative power of yoga. Through her dedication to the practice, she has found healing, strength, and inner peace, reclaiming her life with a sense of purpose and vitality that continues to inspire those around her.

Overcoming Adversity: David's Journey

David's journey with yoga is one of perseverance, courage, and transformation in the face of adversity. Born with a rare genetic condition that left him with limited mobility and chronic pain, David faced countless challenges and setbacks throughout his life. Despite the odds stacked against him, he refused to let his condition define him, choosing instead to embrace the practice of yoga as a source of healing and hope.

Through years of dedicated practice and unwavering determination, David discovered a newfound sense of freedom and empowerment within his body and mind. With each breath and movement, he defied the limitations imposed upon him by his condition, cultivating strength, flexibility, and resilience in the face of adversity.

Today, David's life is a testament to the transformative power of yoga to transcend physical limitations and awaken the spirit. Through his unwavering commitment to the practice, he has overcome seemingly insurmountable obstacles with grace and courage, inspiring others to embrace their own inner strength and resilience in the face of adversity.

Cultivating Self-Acceptance and Inner Peace: Maya's Path

Maya's journey with yoga is one of self-discovery, acceptance, and inner peace. Struggling with low self-esteem and body image issues, Maya spent years trapped in a cycle of self-doubt and negative self-talk, unable to see her own worth and beauty. Frustrated and exhausted by her inner turmoil, she turned to yoga as a path to healing and self-discovery.

Through the practice of yoga, Maya began to cultivate a deeper sense of self-acceptance and compassion towards herself. With each breath and movement, she learned to quiet the critical voice within her mind, replacing it with a sense of love and acceptance for herself just as she is. Through mindfulness and self-reflection, she discovered a newfound sense of inner peace and serenity that had eluded her for so long.

Today, Maya's life is a testament to the transformative power of yoga to heal the body, calm the mind, and awaken the spirit. Through her journey of self-discovery and self-acceptance, she has found a sense of peace and wholeness that radiates from within, inspiring others to embrace their inherent worth and beauty with love and compassion.

The personal stories of Sarah, David, Maya, and countless others serve as powerful reminders of the transformative power of yoga to heal, empower, and awaken the spirit. Through their journeys of self-discovery and transformation, these individuals have found healing, strength, and inner peace amidst life's challenges and adversities. Their stories inspire us to embrace the practice of yoga as a path to self-discovery, healing, and transformation, inviting us to embark on our journey of inner exploration and growth with courage, grace, and compassion. As we cultivate mindfulness, self-compassion, and inner peace through the practice of yoga, may we discover the profound and lasting transformation that awaits us on the path of self-discovery and self-realization.

8.2 Advice for Sustaining a Lifelong Yoga Practice

Maintaining a lifelong yoga practice requires dedication, commitment, and a deep sense of connection to the practice. In this chapter, we will explore valuable advice and insights from experienced yogis who have sustained their practice over many years, navigating the ebbs and flows of life with grace and resilience. Drawing upon their wisdom and expertise, we will uncover practical tips, strategies, and principles for sustaining a lifelong yoga practice that nourishes the body, mind, and spirit, empowering individuals to thrive on and off the mat.

1. Cultivate Consistency and Routine

Set Realistic Goals: Establish realistic goals for your yoga practice that align with your lifestyle, schedule, and commitments. Start with small, manageable goals and gradually increase the frequency and duration of your practice over time.

Create a Routine: Incorporate yoga into your daily or weekly routine by designating specific times and spaces for practice. Consistency is key to sustaining a lifelong practice, so make it a priority to show up on the mat regularly, even on days when motivation is low.

2. Listen to Your Body and Honor Your Limits

Practice Self-Compassion: Listen to your body and honor its signals and limitations with kindness and compassion. Avoid pushing yourself into poses that feel uncomfortable or unsafe, and modify or skip poses as needed to protect your body from injury.

Focus on Quality over Quantity: Prioritize the quality of your practice over the quantity of poses or duration of sessions. Pay attention to how your body feels in each pose and adjust your practice accordingly to ensure that it serves your unique needs and intentions.

3. Embrace Adaptability and Evolution

Be Open to Change: Embrace adaptability and flexibility in your practice, recognizing that it will evolve and change over time. Be open to exploring new styles, techniques, and approaches to yoga that resonate with you at different stages of your life.

Stay Curious and Playful: Approach your practice with a sense of curiosity, exploration, and playfulness. Stay open to new experiences and possibilities, and don't be afraid to step outside of your comfort zone to discover new depths and dimensions of your practice.

4. Cultivate Mindfulness and Presence

Practice Mindful Awareness: Cultivate mindful awareness in your yoga practice by bringing your attention to the present moment with curiosity and non-judgment. Notice sensations, thoughts, and emotions as they arise, and allow them to unfold without attachment or aversion.

Breathe Deeply: Use the breath as a tool for cultivating mindfulness and presence in your practice. Focus on deep, conscious breathing to anchor your awareness in the present moment and connect with the rhythm of your body and breath.

5. Find Community and Support

Connect with Like-Minded Practitioners: Seek out community and support from like-minded practitioners who share your passion for yoga. Join classes, workshops, or online communities to connect with others, share experiences, and draw inspiration from the collective wisdom of the group.

Seek Guidance from Teachers: Seek guidance and support from experienced yoga teachers who can offer personalized instruction, feedback, and encouragement to support your growth and development on the mat.

6. Embrace Yoga off the Mat

Integrate Yoga into Daily Life: Embrace the principles and teachings of yoga off the mat by integrating mindfulness, compassion, and presence into your daily life. Practice yoga in action by embodying its values and principles in your interactions with others and your engagement with the world around you.

Cultivate a Holistic Lifestyle: Embrace a holistic approach to health and well-being by incorporating yoga into all aspects of your life, including nutrition, sleep, stress management, and self-care practices. Nurture your body, mind, and spirit with practices that nourish and support your overall well-being.

Sustaining a lifelong yoga practice requires intention, dedication, and a deep commitment to self-care and self-discovery. By cultivating consistency, adaptability, mindfulness, and community support, individuals can nourish and sustain their practice throughout a lifetime, experiencing the transformative power of yoga to heal, empower, and awaken the body, mind, and spirit. As you embark on your journey of sustaining a lifelong yoga practice, may you embrace these principles with love, compassion, and a sense of curiosity and adventure, discovering the joy and vitality that await you on the path of yoga.

8.3 Insights on Embracing Aging with Grace and Acceptance

Aging is a natural and inevitable part of life's journey, yet it often comes with its own set of challenges and uncertainties. In this chapter, we will explore valuable insights and perspectives on embracing aging with grace, acceptance, and wisdom. Drawing upon the wisdom of seasoned yogis, spiritual teachers, and experts in the field of aging, we will uncover practical advice, inspirational stories, and transformative practices for navigating the journey of aging with grace and dignity, empowering individuals to embrace each stage of life with openness, resilience, and inner peace.

Embracing the Wisdom of Aging

Aging is not just a process of physical decline; it is also a journey of self-discovery, growth, and transformation. As we age, we have the opportunity to cultivate wisdom, compassion, and acceptance towards ourselves and others. By embracing the wisdom of aging, we can navigate life's challenges with grace and resilience, embracing each moment with gratitude and presence.

Cultivating Self-Compassion and Acceptance

As we age, our bodies may change, and our abilities may diminish, but our inherent worth and value remain unchanged. Cultivating self-compassion and acceptance allows us to embrace the aging process with grace and dignity, acknowledging and honoring the beauty and wisdom that come with each passing year. By embracing our imperfections and limitations, we can cultivate a deeper sense of self-acceptance and peace, freeing ourselves from the burden of unrealistic expectations and judgments.

Finding Joy and Fulfillment in Every Stage of Life

Aging is not a destination; it is a journey that unfolds over time, presenting us with new opportunities for growth, connection, and fulfillment. By embracing each stage of life with openness and curiosity, we can discover joy, meaning, and purpose in every moment. Whether we are in the prime of youth or the wisdom of old age, there is beauty and richness to be found in every stage of life, inviting us to savor each moment and embrace the fullness of our experience.

Letting Go of Attachments and Expectations

As we age, we may face the challenge of letting go of attachments and expectations that no longer serve us. Whether it is the pursuit of external validation, the fear of aging, or the pressure to conform to societal norms, letting go of attachments allows us to embrace the present moment with openness and freedom. By releasing the grip of attachment, we can cultivate a deeper sense of peace and contentment, allowing life to unfold naturally and effortlessly.

Nurturing Connections and Relationships

As we age, the quality of our connections and relationships becomes increasingly important. Cultivating meaningful connections with loved ones, friends, and community members enriches our lives and provides us with a sense of belonging and support. By nurturing relationships built on love, compassion, and mutual respect, we can navigate the challenges of aging with grace and dignity, knowing that we are supported and valued by those who matter most to us.

Embracing Change and Adaptability

Aging is a process of constant change and adaptation, requiring us to embrace the ebb and flow of life with grace and resilience. By cultivating a mindset of flexibility and adaptability, we can navigate life's transitions with ease and confidence, embracing new opportunities for growth and learning along the way. Whether it is adjusting to physical changes, career transitions, or shifting roles and responsibilities, embracing change allows us to embrace the fullness of life with an open heart and mind.

Aging is a journey of self-discovery, growth, and transformation that unfolds throughout a lifetime. By embracing the wisdom of aging, cultivating self-compassion and acceptance, finding joy and fulfillment in every stage of life, letting go of attachments and expectations, nurturing connections and relationships, and embracing change and adaptability, we can navigate the journey of aging with grace, dignity, and inner peace. As we embrace each moment with gratitude and presence, may we discover the beauty and richness of life in all its stages, embracing the journey of aging with an open heart and mind.

Conclusion:

In this book, we have explored the transformative power of yoga in maintaining youthful vitality and flexibility throughout your lifetime. Through the wisdom of experienced practitioners, scientific research, and practical insights, we have uncovered the profound benefits of integrating yoga into your daily life to nurture your body, mind, and spirit.

Yoga is more than just a physical practice; it is a holistic system that encompasses breath, movement, mindfulness, and self-awareness. By incorporating yoga into your routine, you can cultivate physical strength, flexibility, and balance, while also promoting mental clarity, emotional well-being, and spiritual growth.

Throughout these pages, we have delved into the various aspects of yoga practice, from gentle poses for beginners to advanced postures for enhancing flexibility, from breathing techniques for stress reduction to meditation practices for clarity and focus. We have explored the ways in which yoga can support joint health and mobility, mental well-being, and overall vitality, helping you to age gracefully and embrace each stage of life with grace and acceptance.

But beyond the physical benefits, yoga offers something deeper—a path to self-discovery, self-acceptance, and self-transformation. Through the practice of yoga, you can cultivate a deeper connection to yourself and the world around you, finding peace, joy, and fulfillment in each moment.

As you embark on your journey with yoga, remember that the key to staying young is not just about maintaining a youthful appearance, but about nurturing your body, mind, and spirit with love, compassion, and intention. Whether you are young or old, beginner or experienced practitioner, yoga offers something for everyone—a pathway to health, happiness, and wholeness.

So, embrace the practice of yoga with an open heart and mind. Allow yourself to explore, experiment, and evolve on your mat and in your life. And above all, remember that the true essence of youth lies not in the passing of time, but in the richness of experience, the depth of connection, and the boundless potential for growth and renewal that yoga offers us all.

May your journey with yoga be filled with joy, vitality, and wonder. And may you stay forever young in body, mind, and spirit, as you continue to discover the infinite possibilities that await you on the path of yoga.

Namaste.